Pestilence in Medieval and Early Modern English Literature

Medieval History and Culture
Volume 23

STUDIES IN

MEDIEVAL HISTORY AND CULTURE

edited by
Francis G. Gentry
Professor of German
Pennsylvania State University

A ROUTLEDGE SERIES

Other Books in This Series:

Marriage Fictions in Old French Secular Narratives, 1170–1250
A Critical Re-evaluation of the Courtly Love Debate
Keith A. Nicklaus

Where Troubadours Were Bishops
The Occitania of Folc of Marseille (c. 1150–1231)
Nichole M. Schulman

John Cassian and the Reading of Egyptian Monastic Culture
Steven D. Driver

Choosing Not to Marry
Women and Autonomy in the Katherine Group
Julie Hassel

Feminine Figurae
Representations of Gender in Religious Texts by Medieval German Women Writers
Rebecca L.R. Garber

Bodies of Pain
Suffering in the Works of Hartmann von Aue
Scott E. Pincikowski

The Literal Sense and the Gospel of John in Late Medieval Commentary and Literature
Mark Hazard

The Reproductive Unconscious in Late Medieval and Early Modern England
Jennifer Wynne Hellwarth

Mystical Language of Sense in the Later Middle Ages
Gordon Rudy

Fair and Varied Forms
Visual Textuality in Medieval Illustrated Manuscripts
Mary C. Olson

Queens in the Cult of the French Renaissance Monarchy
Public Law, Royal Ceremonial, and Political Discourse in the History of Regency Government, 1484–1610
Elizabeth A. McCartney

The Contested Theological Authority of Thomas Aquinas
The Controversies between Hervaeus Natalis and Durandus of St. Pourçain
Elizabeth Lowe

Body and Sacred Place in Medieval Europe, 1100–1389
Dawn Marie Hayes

Women of the Humiliati
A Lay Religious Order in Medieval Civic Life
Sally Mayall Brasher

Consuming Passions
The Uses of Cannibalism in Late Medieval and Early Modern Europe
Merrall Llewelyn Price

Literary Hybrids
Cross-dressing, Shapeshifting, and Indeterminacy in Medieval and Modern French Narrative
Erika E. Hess

The King's Two Maps
Cartography and Culture in Thirteenth-Century England
Daniel Birkholz

Pestilence in Medieval and Early Modern English Literature

Bryon Lee Grigsby

Routledge
New York & London

Published in 2004 by
Routledge
29 West 35th Street
New York, NY 10001
www.routledge-ny.com

Published in Great Britain by
Routledge
11 New Fetter Lane
London EC4P 4EE
www.routledge.co.uk

Routledge is an imprint of the Taylor and Francis Group.
Printed in the United States of America on acid-free paper.

10 9 8 7 6 5 4 3 2

Library of Congress Cataloging-in-Publication Data

Grigsby, Bryon Lee.
Pestilence in Medieval and early modern English literature / by Bryon Lee Grigsby.
p. cm. — (Medieval history and culture; v. 23)
Includes bibliographical references and index.
ISBN 0-415-96822-4 (hardcover : alk. paper)
1. English literature—Middle English, 1100–1500—History and criticism. 2. Medicine in literature. 3. English literature—Early modern, 1500–1700—History and criticism. 4. Literature and medicine—Great Britain—History. 5. Epidemics—Great Britain—History. 6. Diseases—Great Britain—History. 7. Medicine—Great Britain—History. 8. Plague—Great Britain—History. 9. Diseases in literature. 10. Plague in literature. I. Title. II. Series.
PR275.M4G75 2003
820.9'3561—dc22

2003014369

Dedicated to my family:

Henry and Marie Dieckman,

Les and Tina Marie Grigsby

and

Carolyn Coulson-Grigsby and Eliza Marie Grigsby

Series Editor Foreword

Far from providing just a musty whiff of yesteryear, research in Medieval Studies enters the new century as fresh and vigorous as never before. Scholars representing all disciplines and generations are consistently producing works of research of the highest caliber, utilizing new approaches and methodologies. Volumes in the Medieval History and Culture series will include studies on individual works and authors of Latin and vernacular literatures, historical personalities and events, theological and philosophical issues, and new critical approaches to medieval literature and culture.

Momentous changes have occurred in Medieval Studies in the past thirty years in teaching as well as in scholarship. Thus the goal of the Medieval History and Culture series is to enhance research in the field by providing an outlet for monographs by scholars in the early stages of their careers on all topics related to the broad scope of Medieval Studies, while at the same time pointing to and highlighting new directions that will shape and define scholarly discourse in the future.

Francis G. Gentry

Contents

Acknowledgments

I owe a great deal of thanks to a variety of people who fostered my interest in medicine and literature. I first have to thank the New York State Parks and Recreation, specifically Lake Tiorati, for supplying me with a summer job for thirteen years and for the start of my practical medical experience including vehicle extrication, drowning, minor and major first aid, emergency child births, and others. Staff members who have always supported me and furthered my knowledge both as a human being and as a First Responder include Oliver Schreiber, Peter Hechler, Alison Esposito, Dan and Cathi Steinberg, Debbie Hoffman, William and Pat Moore, Scott Richardson, Paul Gordon, Lori Vesely, and Nicole Gulliver. The good times at Tiorati by far outweigh the bad and the traumatic, thanks to all of you.

As for my academic career, I had the fortune and pleasure to work with two very caring professors from Moravian College. I need to thank Dr. Robert Burcaw, my mentor and friend, who continues to fascinate me with his energy about teaching and conviction that literature is about life. It is my hope that I can be half the teacher he was to me. I also have to thank Dr. Carole Brown, who introduced me to Chaucer and to the Middle Ages, at eight o'clock in the morning, spring semester my senior year.

At Wake Forest University, I continued my study of the Middle Ages under two exceptional professors and scholars, Dr. Gillian Overing and Dr. Gail Sigal. Through these professors, I was introduced to Dr. Allen Frantzen whose presentation on a Marxist reading of Chaucer's *Troilus and Criseyde* impressed me to the point that I wanted to be his student.

I owe Allen Frantzen a huge debt, not only for directing my book, but also for being a great and supportive teacher. Whatever scholarship I am able to produce is because of the high standards he has for his graduate students and their studies. I also need to thank Allen for encouraging me to study and write about images of the body in literature, which eventually led to my work on medieval medicine.

I also want to thank Dr. Jo Hays who not only worked on my book, but also was kind enough to do an independent study with me on the History of Medicine; Dr. James Biester who taught me much about Renaissance Literature and Rhetoric; and Dr. Carol Everest, from The King's University College, who agreed to be an outside reader. I thank her for her friendship and scholarship. I would also like to thank Dr. Steve Harris, my friend, editor, and fishing buddy, who made Chicago more enjoyable through rented movies, Jim Beam, and good conversation. Drs. Lachlan and Patricia Peeke were always present to put graduate studies into perspective, and I need to thank them for many nights of counseling and support. From the academic field, I would like to thank the faculty and administration of Centenary College for all their advice and support, particularly Dr. Ken Hoyt, Dr. Angela Elliott, Dr. John Holt, Dr. Debra Fleming, Dr. Ed Barboni, and Rev. David Jones. I would also like to thank former and current students who challenge me on a constant basis to be a better scholar and teacher, particularly Rick Godden, who is finishing his doctorate at University of Washington, St. Louis, and Candice Morris, who helped to index this book.

From my family, I need to especially thank my mother, Tina Marie Grigsby, and my father, Leslie Earle Grigsby, without whose financial and emotional support I would have quit long ago. My maternal grandmother and grandfather taught me more about believing in one's self and one's family than I could have ever learned from a book. To Carolyn Coulson-Grigsby, my wife, best friend, and editor, thank you for providing laughter during all the difficult times. You have given to me more than I can ever repay. And finally to Eliza, my daughter, who provides me constant joy as I watch her grow and develop.

If this work has any value, it is due to all those people who supported me. All the errors, however, are purely my own.

Introduction

In *Illness as Metaphor*, Susan Sontag writes, "Illness is the night-side of life, a more onerous citizenship. Everyone who is born holds dual citizenship, in the kingdom of the well and in the kingdom of the sick. Although we all prefer to use only the good passport, sooner or later each of us is obliged, at least for a spell, to identify ourselves as citizens of that other place" (3). In the Middle Ages, this dual citizenship was extremely pronounced, especially in regard to leprosy and bubonic plague. At one moment a person could hold citizenship in the kingdom of the well, and through an alteration in his or her skin's integrity, change citizenship to the kingdom of the lepers. If buboes erupted, the individual gained access to the pestilent kingdom, and often died within a few days. Outsiders stereotyped members of each kingdom, and identified and associated them with the other citizens of that kingdom. These stereotypes often carry moral connotations and resonate with certain social concerns. A modern example might be someone diagnosed with lung cancer. Most people would assume that he or she had been a smoker, and therefore deserved his or her punishment. The moral connection would be that the smoker, unconcerned with his or her health, committed the "sin" of smoking, and the emphasis on this connection between morality and disease reflects our own culture's almost moral obsession with healthy living.

While Sontag has shown that for cancer and AIDS many of these moral associations with illness are medically unfounded, they still exist. More importantly, these moral connections not only function on a metaphoric level, but also operate on a literal level that needs further examination, especially in the medieval period. For example, when a medieval doctor said that plague was caused by usury, he might not be making metaphorical connections to the state of the patient's soul or of society's morality, but might literally have meant that usury causes the plague. As Sontag has shown, epidemic diseases whose means of transmission is unknown are the diseases most susceptible to moral (what I term metaphoric) associations (*Illness*, 58–9). These moral associations are numerous and shifting. This book follows the moral associations connected to leprosy and bubonic plague by medical, theological, and literary communities from the Middle Ages through the Renaissance. I demonstrate how these epidemic diseases raise concerns about an errant society.

This introduction provides the reader with a description of my methodology, a history of scholarship related to this subject, and an outline of each chapter. Historians have worked diligently over the last ten years to provide the information necessary to understand the medieval health system. It is time to examine how this historical analysis informs literature and to recognize that literature is part of a social system that influences people's thoughts and beliefs, even their medical and religious beliefs. I examine medicine as an outgrowth of theology and demonstrate that the moral associations of leprosy and bubonic plague reflect important social concerns of the medieval and Early Modern Periods.

Critics of medieval literature have been slow to respond to the interdisciplinary study of literature and medicine, maintaining boundaries which contemporary theory has long since discarded. The representations of leprosy and bubonic plague in medieval literature are informed by medical and theological beliefs that are not wholly separated by disciplinary boundaries; rather, both fields might be said to work together and to construct discourses that play out in literature. It is my intention to reconstruct the medieval medical and theological discourses that surround leprosy and bubonic plague in order to gain a better awareness of the literature and culture of this period.

Methodology: Social Constructionism

Developed out of a combination of Foucauldian criticism, poststructuralism, and feminism, social constructionism is the most recent addition to the philosophy and sociology of science. From a medical perspective, social constructionists might examine the institutions that disseminate medical information to the population. For example, each one of us knows a certain amount about illness. Some of our knowledge originates from authoritative medical sources, and some comes from general social knowledge, such as family tradition or ethnic belief. Examples of the former include recognition of a heart attack or stroke as well as the knowledge of how to administer CPR. Of the latter, one possible example is the alleged effect of chicken soup on the causes of a cold or flu. It is not the role of a social constructionist to examine the validity of any of these beliefs. A social constructionist does not evaluate or privilege one type of medical belief over another. Instead, social constructionism points to the social forces that developed these ideas about disease. In *Medicine and Culture*, Deborah Lupton writes that social constructionism

> does not necessarily call into question the reality of disease or illness states or bodily experiences, it merely emphasizes that these states and experiences are known and interpreted via social activity and therefore should be examined using cultural and social analysis. According to this perspective, medical knowledge is regarded not as an incremental progression towards a more refined and better knowledge, but as a series of relative constructions that are dependent upon socio-historical settings in which they occur and are constantly negotiated. (11)

A social constructionist cannot limit himself to the medical community in order to gain an understanding of a specific disease; rather he or she must examine other social communities and their discourse of disease in order to gain a complete picture of how specific illnesses are interpreted, and therefore reacted to.

A clear modern example of the scholarly methods used by social constructionists is Paula Treichler's famous article, "AIDS, Homophobia, and Biomedical Discourse: An Epidemic of Signification," which examines the linguistic construction of AIDS as a homosexual disease. Treichler traces the adjectives originally used to describe the organs affected by AIDS, such as the "vulnerable anus," the "fragile urethra," and the "rugged vagina." These phrases and their connotations led both medical doctors and the popular press to declare erroneously: "AIDS isn't a threat to the vast majority of heterosexuals.... It is now—and is likely to remain—largely the fatal price one can pay for anal intercourse" (37). These associations not only gave certain social groups a false sense of security, but also reaffirmed political, social, and moral constructions of modern society that had little to do with the medical facts of HIV or AIDS.

Similar social constructions surrounded medieval diseases, such as leprosy and bubonic plague. Unaware of viruses and bacteria, medieval medical practitioners considered medicine to be a part of theology; the governing assumption being that immoral behavior caused illness. Hence, medical authorities throughout the Middle Ages and into the Renaissance asserted that immoral behavior led to disease and illness. I trace the relationship between medicine and theology in the social construction of medieval diseases and, on that basis, describe what certain illnesses can mean in literature.

History of Scholarship

There is very little literary scholarship on the medieval relationship between medicine and literature, and what little there is either deals only with medicine's link to astrology or attempts to construct an evolutionary narrative by which medieval medicine becomes a naïve precursor to modern medicine. While most people would tend to consider medicine to be a science, scholars of medieval literature do not seem to agree. What little work has been done on medieval literature and science has concentrated on Chaucer and his use of astrology. Walter Clyde Curry's *Chaucer and the Medieval Sciences* (1926), has been the best work available to Chaucerians on medieval science and literature. But this work also focuses heavily, almost exclusively, on astrology. In *Approaches to Teaching Chaucer's Canterbury Tales* (1980), Joseph Gibaldi states, "Scholarship devoted to Chaucer and medieval science has increased in recent times to such a degree that a chapter on the subject (written by Chauncey Wood) is included in Rowland's *Companion to Chaucer's Studies*" (26). However, Wood's chapter examines only astrology, and no other medieval sciences. Furthermore, of the eighty-seven sources Wood cites, not one relates to medicine. Obviously there is more to medieval science than star-gazing. Outside the realm of Chaucer and astrology, little work has been done on the relationship between medicine and literature.

Most recently, R. Allen Shoaf published *Chaucer's Body: The Anxiety of Circulation in the Canterbury Tales* (2001). This very informative and learned book treats circulation and infection as metaphors for writing and rhetoric. Shoaf writes, "This book is probably best characterized as an essay in cultural studies, since, necessarily, it combines history, literature, politics, theology, and philosophy in its argument" (8). However, as Shoaf rightly recognizes his work is essentially about Chaucer's rhetoric and how words can and do infect people. It is not about the literal interpretations disease or how the discourse communities of medicine and literature interact.

The Positivist Approach

Only three literary critics–Saul Brody, Barbara Fass Leavy, and Peregrine Horden–have explored the relationship between medicine and literature outside of Chaucer, and two of those works seem to approach the medieval period from a positivistic framework that attempts to see medieval medicine as a primitive form of modern medicine. Brody and Leavy might be said to indulge in positivistic thinking. Saul Brody's 1974 publication, *The Disease of the Soul: Leprosy and Medieval Literature*, is the most highly regarded study on leprosy and literature. This work traces medical, theological, and historical reactions to lepers, devoting one chapter to leprosy in literature from the Anglo-Saxon to modern period. His book is thus a very general study of medieval literary texts and their social context. Given Brody's immense undertaking, he perhaps had little choice but to make tenuous connections between medieval and modern viewpoints of leprosy. This comparison works well as a teaching method to increase interest in the Middle Ages, but it does little to help the medieval scholar understand how people in the Middle Ages understood and constructed disease, because it uses modern interpretations of disease as a paradigm to judge earlier interpretations.

Barbara Fass Leavy's *To Blight with Plague: Studies in a Literary Theme* (1992) "is a study of literary works whose main themes have to do with some form of contagious or pestilential physical disease, and the social or psychological consequences of the illness" (1). Leavy does not attempt "to write a comprehensive history of plague literature"(2); she concentrates on bubonic plague, syphilis, influenza, and AIDS in the literature of the Western canon. "Since this is not primarily a study of sources," she writes, "I have in some instances been content to point out similarities in motifs from work to work without being concerned to establish direct links" (2). Leavy dedicates one chapter to the earliest mentions of plague in post-classical literature (in Chaucer and Boccaccio) and shows their effects on Edgar Allan Poe and Daniel Defoe. Leavy's framework forces her to generalize about the effects of specific diseases during different time periods. While such unavoidably superficial comparison is useful for connecting an earlier culture's treatment of plague to our own treatment of AIDS, it only hints at the varied and multiple interpretations of plague within a specific period. For example, Leavy is interested in demonstrating the tension authors felt between self-preservation and civic duty, but she understandably does not explore how the medical or theological community also informs a tension felt by authors of the Middle Ages.

Peregrine Horden's "Disease, Dragons and Saints in the Dark Ages," published in a 1992 collection entitled *Epidemics and Ideas: Essays on the Historical Perception of Pestilence*, attempts to avoid one of the most common pitfalls of the scholarship regarding disease, "superficial comparativism" between different cultures (47). Horden argues that dragons are often recorded as having pestiferous breath and living in swamps, which could imply a relationship between the dragon and malaria (47). Most critics interpret this connection as symbolic and make connections to other cultures and other time periods. However, Horden treats the relationship between dragons and pestiferous breath literally and connects it to the medical and literary evidence from that community and time.

One of the reasons medieval literary scholars have relied on superficial comparisons and have been slow to investigate the relationship between disease and literature outside a positivistic framework is that medieval historians have only recently started to research the construction of both the medieval medical community and disease on its own terms. In 1986 Nancy Siraisi stated that "in almost all areas of medieval and Renaissance medical history, fundamental work remains to be done" ("Editorial" 392). Medieval historians have attempted to reconstruct the medical system in four ways: the validity of medieval medicine, medieval society's response to the medical community, a rediscovery of previously ignored medical texts, and the role of disease in both the medical and the social communities. A brief critical history of the major works on these four theoretical points will show that historians have been moving from a positivist to a social constructionist framework within which medicine is viewed as part of a social system.

Early scholars of medieval medicine found medieval doctors' theories ridiculous. For example, in *A Short History of Medicine* (1962), Charles Singer found medieval medicine demonstrative of "the wilting mind of the Dark Ages" (31). Singer also believed that medieval medicine, specifically the Anglo-Saxon herbals, "lacked any rational element which might mark the beginnings of scientific advance" (qtd. in Cameron 3). More recently, historians such as M. L. Cameron (*Anglo-Saxon Medicine* [1993]) and John Riddle (*Contraception and Abortion from the Ancient World to the Renaissance* [1992]) have attempted to validate medieval medicine in light of modern medicine. By analyzing common herbals, both Cameron and Riddle have found a few recipes that have therapeutic merit. However, Singer, Cameron, and Riddle approach medieval medicine from a positivistic framework that attempts to see modern medicine foreshadowed in medieval medicine. Singer attempted to reinterpret the ideas of medieval medicine in light of modern scientific discoveries. Not finding a way to accomplish this reinterpretation, he dismisses the entire corpus. Similarly, Cameron and Riddle attempt to validate medieval medicine by showing that the roots of our modern pharmacology can be found in ancient herbals.

The Social Construction of the Medieval Medical Community

Rather than approach the medieval medical community from a positivistic framework in which the medieval doctor is a primitive reflection of our modern doctor, some historians have attempted to evaluate the medieval medical community as part of a social system. The most general work on the reconstruction of the medical system is Siraisi's *Medieval and Early Renaissance Medicine: An Introduction to Knowledge and Practice* (1990), which explores the development of medicine in Italy between the mid-twelfth and fifteenth centuries. This work greatly expanded on such historical works as Charles Talbot's *Medicine in Medieval England* (1965), Edward Kealey's *Medieval Medicus: A Social History of Anglo-Norman Medicine* (1981), and Katherine Park's *Doctors and Medicine in Early Renaissance Florence* (1985). According to Siraisi, medicine infiltrates many aspects of medieval culture: "[I]n the complex society of the late Middle Ages and early Renaissance, the spectrum of medical practitioners encompassed men and women, laity and clergy, learned scholastics and illiterate herbalists, and institutions connected with medicine including both guilds and universities" (ix). Scholars are moving toward a better understanding of medieval society because they no longer deal with medieval medicine as an isolated discipline, but as part of a social system which involved a myriad of institutions.

Two medieval historians have attempted to contextualize medicine within a specific period. In *Medicine Before the Plague: Practitioners in the Crown of Aragon, 1285–1345* (1993), Michael McVaugh complains that "historians of medieval science, even more than their counterparts studying other periods, have been slow to explore the general context of their subject, and have concentrated instead upon understanding and communicating the learned natural-philosophical texts that embody so much of it" (ix). McVaugh reconstructs the health care system of medieval Spain to see how common people responded not only to illness and disease but also to learned and empiric medicine. Thus we see that historians are demonstrating that medieval medicine varies at different periods and in different locations, focusing on specific periods and specific regions in order to avoid unwarranted generalizations common to earlier criticism.

For the purposes of this book, I examine mainly works written in the English vernacular from the fourteenth through the sixteenth centuries. There are only a few historical works that pay close attention to medicine in England during the fourteenth and fifteenth centuries. Robert Gottfried's *Epidemic Disease in Fifteenth-Century England* (1978) explores the effects of plague on East Anglia through the fifteenth century, paying particular attention to wills from that area and time period. Gottfried's work is specific in both medical and geographic scope. Carole Rawcliffe's *Medicine and Society in Later Medieval England* (1995) provides a more general look at all aspects of English medicine in the fourteenth and fifteenth centuries. Rawcliffe's work provides much fundamental information about the nature of medical studies, the methods of treatment, and the development of a medical hierarchy. Rawcliffe identifies the problems many modern historians encounter when trying to explain medieval medicine:

> The idea of separating ... the treating of physical symptoms without addressing the spiritual malaise of the sufferer would have seemed both profane and pointless. Historians of medieval medicine can hardly avoid making such an anachronistic distinction, and in concentrating almost exclusively upon the treatment of the body the rest of this book illuminates just one corner of a far broader canvas. (25)

Rawcliffe's illumination does extend beyond the body, however, and examines the creation and contextualization of the medical hierarchy, paying particular attention to the work of women in the medical field.

While Rawcliffe is interested in how women functioned in the medical community of the Later Middle Ages, other scholars have attempt to examine how medical theories shaped social beliefs about gender. Joan Cadden's *Meanings of Sex Difference in the Middle Ages* (1993) expands on the groundbreaking work of Danielle Jacquart's and Claude Thomasset's *Sexuality and Medicine in the Middle Ages* (1985) to explore how medical texts interacted with religious beliefs about gender and sexuality. In Jacquart and Thomasset's work, the authors used medical and literary works to trace the developments of the conception of gender, courtly love, and venereal disease. Using the same primary sources, Cadden examines "the question of differences between males and females"(8). According to Cadden, "The plot of this account ... does not consist in the discovery of the essence of medieval views on sex difference and the logic of their relation to a gender system; instead it consists in the unfolding of relations among various distinct but overlapping theories, values, and interests" (10). In other words, Cadden articulates a theory in which theology, literature, and medicine inform gender constructions.

Social Construction: Disciplinary Boundaries

Along similar theoretical lines, Darrel W. Amundsen's *Medicine, Society, and Faith in the Ancient and Medieval Worlds* (1996) defends the notion that medicine and theology were unified disciplines. Amundsen's book is a collection of essays, and he recognizes that he has many themes, but two themes loom largest: "(1) the disputed boundaries of Christianity and medicine (and the question of the propriety of medicine for Christians); (2) respect for human life, that is, a principle of sanctity of human life (including the duty to treat or to attempt to sustain the life of the ill)" (xi). Amundsen sees medicine as a product of both theology and philosophy, a product that can be traced back to Greco-Roman and Early Christian society. He also examines the complex moral issues doctors faced during outbreaks of both bubonic plague and syphilis.

Since medical information can be found in a variety of non-medical sources, historians have found it difficult to contextualize medicine within medieval society. The contributors to *Manuscript Sources of Medieval Medicine* (1995), edited by Margaret R. Schleissner, demonstrate that various kinds of works—from calendars to handbooks—contain different forms of medical information. In "Multitudes of Middle English Medical Manuscripts, or the Englishing of Science and Medicine," Linda Ehrsam Voights investigates numerous manuscripts in the English vernacular that still need to be fully explored. Voights has discovered more than 7,500 Middle English texts on both medicine and science, many of them unpublished. In *Healing and Society in Medieval England* (1991), Faye Marie Getz has published one important vernacular manuscript, the pharmaceutical writings of Gilbertus Anglicus. However, fundamental work still needs to be done on medieval medical manuscripts, especially the publication, analysis, and transcription of vernacular works of the later Middle Ages.

Social Constructionism: Disease

Two historians have attempted to contextualize the medical system by analyzing both medical and social responses to a wide range of health problems and diseases. One of the best works on nosology (the classification of disease) and the history of disease is the 1989 translation of Mirko Grmek's *Diseases in the Ancient Greek World*. First published in 1983, this book traces diseases from the Greek and Roman worlds through the Middle Ages and Renaissance. Relying on paleopathology, Grmek argues against critics who suggest that certain modern diseases did not exist in earlier societies and provides statistical evidence for the presence of diseases like leprosy, tuberculosis, syphilis, hyperostosis, anemia, and malaria. Grmek is concerned only with proving the existence of certain illnesses, not with analyzing the popular responses or beliefs about them. Grmek is important to social constructionists because he validates the observation that modern terminology for certain diseases fits a past culture's terminology, therefore allowing social constructionists the ability to talk about the construction of the same disease in different time periods. Other historians are interested in both the civic and medical responses to illness. In *Health, Disease, and Healing in Medieval Culture* (1992), edited by Sheila Campbell, Bert Hall, and David Klausner, the contributors examine general and specific illnesses and how they relate to both medieval and modern societies.

Both bubonic plague and leprosy have prompted a fair amount of scholarship on the causes of disease and the medical community's response. Robert Gottfried's *The Black Death: Natural and Human Disaster in Medieval Europe* (1983) examines the ecological events that contributed to the Black Death, the social and economic changes that occurred as a result of depopulation, and the history of bubonic plague scholarship. Other scholars, such as J. F. D. Shrewsbury, argue that bubonic plague did not have the destructive power that most historians give it. In *History of the Bubonic Plague in the British Isles* (1970), Shrewsbury states:

> [T]he contemporary records demonstrate conclusively that over the country as a whole there was no collapse of agriculture, no disruption of the economic life of the nation, for the simple reason that bubonic plague was biologically incapable of destroying under the social conditions existing in fourteenth-century England as much as 20 per cent of its population of some 4 million persons *of all ages*. (123)

Shrewsbury uses a variety of historical documents in an effort to construct the social problems medieval people faced during and after the bubonic plague. Other diseases also influenced the mortality rate; however, most historians, like Shrewsbury, believe that the bubonic plague was a major force in the economic, agricultural, and social lives of medieval people.

More recently, in "Facing the Black Death: Perceptions and Reactions of University Medical Practitioners" (1994), Jon Arrizabalaga examines how medical authorities influenced civil law on issues such as quarantine and decontamination. Finally, in *The Burdens of Disease* (1998), Jo Hays explores a variety of epidemic diseases, including bubonic plague, in order to investigate "the impact of disease on Western civilization, especially in particular episodes or periods in which one disease seemed unusually formidable" (7). Hays's work discusses diseases such as bubonic plague, leprosy, syphilis, tuberculosis, and AIDS. Even though Hays is interested in post-Enlightenment medicine, I am indebted to his work because he successfully combines "pathological reality" with "social constructionism" in order to demonstrate that epidemic disease "affects individuals as well as civilizations" (2).

Leprosy is the most famous disease in which members of the civil, medical, and theological communities advocated quarantine for those suffering from the disease. Besides Saul Brody's work, Peter Richards's *The Medieval Leper* (1977) adds to the scholarship on leprosy by examining the historical relationship between medieval leper colonies and the seventeenth-century lepers of Åland. Richards finds that many of the medieval beliefs concerning uncleanness remained with lepers in later periods. Richards's work, like Brody's, constructs the social interpretation of leprosy from a positivistic framework by producing a narrative in which certain medieval notions about leprosy can be traced to the present day.

Even more recently, in *Epidemics and History: Disease, Power, and Imperialism* (1997), Sheldon Watts argues that medical and political responses to epidemics are tools of imperial forces. Watts, too, is guilty of superficial comparativism by attempting to construct a global narrative for epidemic diseases, from plague, leprosy, and syphilis to smallpox, cholera, yellow fever, and malaria. In all, Watts's book spans six centuries, numerous diseases, and a variety of geographical locations; consequently, his assessments of the Middle Ages are general and broad. However, Watts does point out that disease can be considered within a social context:

> Though epidemiological contexts differed, very often the elite would claim that the disease targeted one particular set of people while leaving others alone. Arrived at through a complex of cultural filters, this perception was part of what I term the disease Construct (as in Construct leprosy, or Construct yellow fever). In establishing official responses, this Construct determined what—if anything—should be done in an attempt to limit disease transmission. (xv)

While Watts's work on disease construction is intent on proving the colonialist motivations of imperial nations, one could also examine the construct to elucidate a specific country's social fears. Watts is correct in assuming that when one is faced with an epidemic disease one tries to find those that caused it. But the agents of the disease are not always members of other nations or religions. Sometimes medical, theological, and civil authorities found moral behaviors within their own people to be both reprehensible and the perceived cause of disease. Therefore by examining the morality these authorities believed caused the disease, one is able to identify the larger social fears present within the society of that time period.

Now that much of the fundamental scholarship has been undertaken, medieval historians have started to move away from positivistic thinking that seeks to interpret medieval medicine as either backwards and worthless or as a primitive evolutionary aspect of modern medicine. Positivistic thinking of this kind either leads to outright rejection of evidentiary material or simplifies that material in order to see reflections of the medieval in the modern. These reflections or superficial comparisons are valuable pedagogical tools that interest undergraduate students learning about the Middle Ages or the history of medicine; however, they do little to further our understanding of the people of the Middle Ages and their social systems. For example, medieval and modern medicine differ most markedly in the interpretation of disease. Disease for medieval doctors is caused by a humoral imbalance, whereas modern doctors believe that most diseases are caused by an invading pathogen. For the medieval doctor, disease is caused by an internal problem, but for the modern doctor, disease is caused by external situations. The difference between internal and external causes for disease will dramatically change the medical interpretations as well as the social interpretations of people with specific diseases. Only by reconstructing the medieval medical interpretation of health and disease can one begin to understand the uses of similar ideas in other social discourses.

More recent scholars investigate medieval medical beliefs as a part of a social construction that influenced medieval society. Because historians have produced the fundamental work necessary to understand and evaluate the medieval medical system, one can now examine how the medical system fit into larger social frameworks and discourses. Medieval medicine was not an isolated part of the society. Instead, doctors participated in a social system that influenced and was influenced by other discourses, such as theology and literature. Only by using what historians have recently reconstructed can one begin to see the influence medicine had on other discourses and on the interpretation of disease.

Overview of Chapters

This book focuses on two diseases, leprosy and bubonic plague, although I will also examine syphilis as a disease that changed leprosy's social construction in the Renaissance. The aims of this book are to reconstruct the belief system surrounding these diseases, to demonstrate how this system changed over time, and to explore the ways literary authors used this information about disease. These two diseases are unified by the moral interpretations people made. The moral associations people attached to leprosy were clearly defined by biblical sources and believed by medical personal. The associations were primarily from the category of spiritual sin, namely, Pride, Envy, Wrath, and Anger. Since leprosy was difficult to contract and since the numbers of lepers declined in the later Middle Ages, beliefs connecting lepers and morality survived.

When the bubonic plague struck, however, doctors and priests attempted to construct a similar moral explanation for the presence of this disease. This time, because of the mass numbers of fatalities, the moral connection between sin and disease was too difficult to make. Doctors and theologians were left to assume that the plague came because of the all-encompassing sin of Pride. Eventually people realized that this disease was not the end of the world and began dealing with the disease in a practical manner, primarily by providing readers with guidance about ways to avoid contagion and to treat those infected. One can read the change in the interpretation of disease as a movement from divine to human control. In other words, with the advent of bubonic plague, people at first saw God as the reason for this plague, much as they had done with the construction of leprosy. Eventually, people realized that they could take control of the disease and live with it by protecting themselves.

When syphilis struck the people of the Renaissance, the first interpretations were similar to those of medieval leprosy owing largely to the fact that one skin disease is like another. However, syphilis had clear moral associations because the disease affected sexual organs, thereby implying that the disease punished those guilty of lechery. With this interpretation, leprosy gained some of the sexual associations that were being ascribed to syphilis. Consequently, moral connections commonly associated with leprosy moved from the spiritual to carnal sins, primarily sexual sins. Again, a change is seen where the interpretation of disease moves from the belief that only God controls disease to a belief that man's actions are responsible for illness.

The first chapter of this book explores the way Greco-Roman medicine was Christianized by early Church leaders. I trace the development of medicine as an aspect of natural philosophy, from medicine's Greco-Roman roots to the Middle Ages. I explain the development of humoral therapy, the relationship between microcosm and macrocosm, and the similarities between doctors and priests. This historical background is important in order to understand a medical system that saw the body as affected by a person's morality and illness as representative of an individual's or a community's immorality.

The second chapter gives a historical overview of leprosy, bubonic plague, and syphilis, from both modern and medieval viewpoints. For leprosy, I use the medical writings of Lanfrank, Henri de Mondeville, and John Arderne and theological claims about illness found in the *Fasciculus Morum* and in penitential manuals. I pay particular attention to the sin(s) that the doctors or priests associated with leprosy. For bubonic plague, I provide a historical narrative of the latest works to examine the construction of the disease. I also explore some contemporary medical and theological beliefs concerning the disease in order to show how the same interpretations that were applied to leprosy were also being used for bubonic plague. The introduction of syphilis into European society during the Renaissance changed the moral associations of leprosy. Since syphilis damages the skin much like leprosy, and since Renaissance people knew that syphilis was transmitted primarily through sex, medical and theological authors connected leprosy to lust. The end of this chapter examines how these writers connected syphilis to others sins more commonly associated with leprosy, but eventually narrowed the field to just one sin, lechery.

Chapter three explores how the connection between sin and disease functions in literary works. For leprosy, I examine the medieval romance *Amis and Amiloun*, Chaucer's *The Summoner's Tale*, John Gower's *Confessio Amantis* and *Mirrour de l'Omme*, and Robert Henryson's *The Testament of Cresseid*. Most scholars have focused on the relationship between leprosy and the sin of lechery. However, one historian, Luke Demaitre, has argued that fourteenth-century doctors did not regularly believe leprosy to be either contagious or venereal. Following Demaitre, I argue that the relationship between sexuality and leprosy is a modern, not a medieval, construction. While it is true that medieval medical doctors believed that victims of leprosy suffered from insatiable sexuality, they found that the desire for sex occurred only after the presence of the disease. In other words, insatiable sexuality is an effect, not a cause, of leprosy. Causes of leprosy in both medieval literature and medical manuals vary greatly, but the Old Testament, primarily the Book of Leviticus, provides the authoritative belief that leprosy was a punishment for simony and envy. Also, leprosy, especially in literature, is not a disease that punishes collective transgressions, but one that punishes individuals who have sinned. Consequently, there is no need in medicine, theology, or literature to justify or explain the punishment of innocent victims, because all individuals who get leprosy must be guilty of sin.

In chapter four, I compare the medical and theological responses concerning bubonic plague to William Langland's *Piers Plowman*, pageants from the York and N-town *Corpus Christi* plays, and Chaucer's *The Pardoner's Prologue* and *Tale*. These works include the first mention of bubonic plague in English literature. By examining the first moral connections made to this disease, these works provide the groundwork for understanding how the interpretation of the disease changed over time. For the primary medical and religious works on the Black Death, I rely on Rosemary Horrox's *The Black Death*, which collects the first religious, literary, and medical responses to the disease from both the British Isles and the Continent.

Since plague is not an event that occurred at one point in history and then vanished, but rather an event that recurred throughout time, my fifth chapter examines how other periods construct plague discourses, discourses which find their roots in medieval thought. In chapter five, I continue my discussion of this plague discourse by interpreting two rarely examined works, John Lydgate's "A Dietary, and a Doctrine for Pestilence" and William Bullein's *A Dialogue Against the Feuer Pestilence*. In every period, people believe that plague highlights a weakness in society. By examining the construction of a plague discourse, one can also examine what authors perceived to be the social and human weaknesses of the time. Furthermore, as people deal with a new disease, they first construct it as "the other" and often blame marginalized groups for the disease's presence. As the disease remains with a society, it becomes part of its fabric, and people begin to deal with the disease more rationally, intelligently, and humanely.

Chapter six examines the use of leprosy in the Renaissance by literary authors. In this period, two different interpretative frameworks developed regarding this disease. On one hand, literary authors continued the medieval association of leprosy with spiritual sins, but, on the other hand, they developed a new line of thought in which leprosy was linked to syphilis and the carnal sins. For the medieval line of thought, I explore Francis Bacon's *Advancement of Learning*, Edmund Spenser's *The Fairie Queen*, and Girolamo Fracastoro's *Syphilis*. For the association of leprosy with syphilis and lechery, I examine William Shakespeare's *Timon of Athens*, *Anthony and Cleopatra*, *2 Henry VI*, and *Henry V*; Ben Jonson's *Volpone*; and John Ford's *'Tis Pity She's a Whore*. Shakespeare's works demonstrate a shift from a nonsexual moral association to a sexual association that is then used by Jonson and Ford. Prior to Shakespeare, the medieval moral associations with leprosy were most common.

As people struggle with AIDS, some authors have seen reflections in the mirror of the Middle Ages. Works like Tony Kushner's *Angels in America*, Ann Benson's *The Plague Tales*, and Anne Rice's *Servant of the Bones* attempt to connect bubonic plague to AIDS, especially in relation to social responses. What each of these authors demonstrates is that while medical technology has made remarkable advances since the Middle Ages, communal responses to infected people have not changed. Whether a social critic is discussing AIDS or bubonic plague, Boccaccio's words still ring true: "They said that the only medicine against the plague striken was to go away from them. Men and women, convinced of this and caring about nothing but themselves, abandoned their own city, their own houses, their dwellings, their relatives, their property, and went abroad or at least to the country of Florence" (3). The association between morality and disease allows the healthy to abandon the sick because it allows them to believe that the sick brought it on themselves.

As people continue to pass from the kingdom of the healthy to the kingdom of the ill, we need to recognize that the passport between these kingdoms is part of a social construction. The moral associations a society applies to the kingdom of the ill demonstrate what people of that time period fear most. By tracking the moral associations of these medieval epidemics, I not only demonstrate the perceived social problems of that time, but also forecast how our own perceptions about AIDS may change as the disease becomes part of the social fabric, as bubonic plague and leprosy did for many centuries of human civilization. AIDS is one of the diseases in which one can hold dual citizenship in both the kingdom of the healthy and ill because modern medicine can make one appear healthy while still being both sick and contagious. Like countries who feel threatened by dual citizenship, we feel threatened by the dual citizenship of PWAs because the boundaries are no longer clearly drawn.

CHAPTER ONE

From *Sophrosyne* to Sin

There are two main reasons why medieval literary critics should reevaluate the role of medicine in literature. The first is that most scholarship about medieval medicine has appeared since 1980; therefore, a lack of material is no longer a valid excuse for misunderstanding medical discourses. The second is that while most of the work about medieval science and literature emphasizes Chaucer and astrology, there is more to science than stargazing. Now that historians know a good deal more about medieval medicine, its relation to society, and its complex role in medieval thought, one can begin to understand how medical discourses interacted with other discourses which in turn shaped social responses to disease. These social responses to disease are influenced by a variety of disciplines, including the medical, theological, and literary.

The best way to explore the interaction of these disciplines is to examine the construction of health from its Greco-Roman roots to its medieval Christianization. Greco-Roman doctors believed in a humoral system where an individual could maintain health through the practice of *sophrosyne* or moderation. *Sophrosyne* was both a mental and physical regimen that was believed to keep the humors balanced. Eventually, the concept of *sophrosyne* was Christianized and immoderation became sin. The relationship between sin and health provided the foundation and the means of interpretation for many authors in the Middle Ages. Throughout this chapter, I will rely on many sources, both primary and secondary, but I am most indebted to the works of Oswei Temkin for providing the foundation of Greco-Roman medicine and the Christianization of that system.

Greco-Roman Medicine

Medieval medicine is neither a precursor to our modern medicine nor a simplistic, primitive system. Rather it is an extremely learned theory that makes sense when one considers the information doctors of the period had to rely on. To do medieval medicine justice, it is necessary to reconstruct the development of this system in relation to health and illness. One must first realize that there are few similarities between medieval and modern medicine, especially in regard to the framework through which each approaches illness.

During the medieval period, the body reflected one's state of health, and medieval doctors relied on the body as text. The body provided medieval doctors with a series of signs and symbols which needed to be read and interpreted in order to provide an effective cure. A modern example of the body being used as text occurs when emergency medical technicians (EMTs) check for unequal pupil size in accidents involving possible head injuries. If one pupil is larger than the other, the EMT suspects a serious head injury, thereby reading and interpreting the injury through the text written in the body. Today, the body as text is rarely used as the only witness to the health of the individual. Instead, medical tests are the means by which health is evaluated (Lupton 98).[1] In most cases, when the body does act as the text, the disease has often progressed very far, making it more difficult to cure.

Medieval doctors had no concept of germs as the cause of illness and no way to test for illness apart from the body itself. Jo Hays writes, "That disease exists 'out there,' and that it invades us, is a view that first gained particular currency in the late nineteenth century, especially because the persuasive power of explanations involving bacteria and viruses made those organisms seem the very essence of disease itself" (3). Medieval doctors approached illness through a markedly different framework than modern doctors do. While the body was known to degenerate with age, medieval doctors believed that a healthy body required a state of harmony or balance. An unhealthy body represented an imbalance, usually identified through a change or sign on the outside of the body, either on the skin or from an excreted fluid, such as urine. Thus the body becomes the text which the doctor needs to interpret in order to first diagnose and then cure. In many ways, we can see a parallel type of interpretation whereby a modern doctor receives a series of numbers from a blood test and produces a diagnosis and treatment for the identified illness. For medieval doctors, the body was the test that needed interpretation.

Lacking any concept of viruses or bacteria as causes of illness, medieval doctors were left to reason that certain behaviors led to illness. There were three types of possible illnesses: those caused by the body's natural degeneration, those the body was predisposed to, and those caused by immoderate living (Temkin, *Hippocrates*, 9). We have a similar system in that we believe that people who smoke, eat red meat, or sunbathe are more prone to cancer and heart disease. We connect these diseases to either a predisposition, such as a hereditary line for breast cancer or heart disease, or to immoderate lifestyle, such as actions that lead to lung disease or liver cancer. While both medieval and modern medicine have a similar emphasis on personal behavior as a cause of illness, medieval medicine's difference lies in the idea that certain sins could cause illnesses. The belief that certain illnesses were caused by specific behavior developed from authoritative Greco-Roman medicine, which was itself eventually influenced and modified by Christian thought.

These medieval notions of disease and morality are not simply metaphors; instead, they were seen as literal truths. Only by understanding the authoritative medical tradition through which doctors learned that immorality caused illness can we begin to see the social construction of disease in a variety of discourses. If, for example, one believes that a certain form of moral transgression causes illness, then the only way to alleviate illness is to correct the moral failings of an individual or of a community. In this sense, literature helps to inform people about the consequences of immorality in the hope that people will renounce sin and thereby help to eliminate the epidemic diseases which threaten to destroy the society.

The connections between morality and illness are not a medieval creation, but are rather part of the heritage of Greco-Roman medicine. Prior to Galen, the Greek medical community was split into three sects: the Empiricists, the Dogmatists, and the Methodists. All three sects continued to have followers through the Middle Ages and beyond; however, the unity Galen created between the Empiricists and Dogmatists had the strongest influence on medieval medicine. Each sect had its own beliefs about the cause of illness. The Empiricists believed that "in the treatment of the sick and similarly in dietary prescriptions, it ought to be possible to dispense with speculation and rely completely on experience" (Temkin, *Galenism*, 15). In this framework, there is no need to learn the theoretical basis for the health of the body; instead, "[t]he successful physician should concentrate on visible symptoms and visible causes and recommend therapy on the basis of past experiences (his own and that of his predecessors) of the efficacy of various remedies" (Lindberg 124).

The Dogmatists, on the other hand, "granted logical arguments a place in medical thought" (Temkin, *Galenism*, 19). This sect believed that not all medical knowledge could be gained through clinical experience, but must be learned through authoritative texts. The Dogmatists relied on a learned tradition and defended the notion of a microcosm and macrocosm (Temkin, *Galenism*, 19). The microcosm consisted of the four bodily humors: blood, phlegm, black bile, and yellow bile. Each of the four humors reflected the elements of the macrocosm: air, water, earth, and fire, respectively. The humors also had a temperature and degrees of moisture. Blood was hot and wet, phlegm was cold and wet, black bile was cold and dry, and yellow bile was hot and dry. According to this theory, when a person became sick, one of the four humors was out of balance. To balance the humors, one needed to take a prescription, usually made from some combination of plants or animals. Doctors categorized all plants and animals by their temperature and moisture. Thus, if a patient's illness was caused by an imbalance of phlegm, which is cold and wet, he or she needed to counteract that humor with its opposite, yellow bile. Therefore, he or she would need to take a prescription made from plants and animals that were hot and dry. According to this system, humans are inherently connected to the natural elements because these elements, not germs, influence health.

Both the Empiricists and the Dogmatists venerated Hippocrates as the central authority on medical knowledge.[2] But by the first century, the Methodist sect, founded by Thessalus, Nero's physician, questioned all authoritative or clinical learning (Temkin, *Galenism*, 31). This sect "rejected both etiological research and experience and inferred directly from the symptoms of disease to the status of the body, which, they thought, was tense or relaxed" (Temkin, *Galenism*, 31–2). Thessalus also boasted that he could "teach medicine in six months, clearly with complete disregard for the ancients" (Temkin, *Galenism*, 32). At the same time that Thessalus was founding the Methodist sect, Galen was combining the central tenets of the Empiricists and Dogmatists. Galen believed that authoritative learning was important but must not be accepted blindly; "rather, [medical authorities] are authorities in as far as they are proved right" through clinical experience (Temkin, *Galenism*, 32). Essentially, Galen saw medicine as a cumulative process in which one studied medical authorities and appended or altered the authoritative corpus through clinical experience.

Galen fought the Methodists because he believed that "they [were] not motivated by love for truth, but by greed and lust and by desire for political power" (Temkin, *Galenism*, 35). Galen's rebuke of the Methodist sect demonstrates the emphasis he placed on morality. According to Galen, the Methodists could not be the preservers of medical truth, for they desired worldly goods, and the desire of worldly goods demonstrates a weak character. For Galen, health results from controlling the passions through *sophrosyne*, or moderation (Temkin, *Galenism*, 37). The control of the passions, both physical and mental, is what becomes Christianized into concepts of sin and redemption. Against the Methodist's desire for worldly goods, Galen argued that his own life was an example of moderate living—he used his father's inheritance to buy only the necessities of life: food, clothing, shelter, and medications (Temkin, *Galenism*, 37). The rest of his money went toward buying books and training stenographers, calligraphers, and students (Temkin, *Galenism*, 37). Galen's argument against the Methodists is a matter of simple logic: if health is the result of moderation, and if the Methodists practice immoderation through the desire for worldly goods, then their ideology cannot be medically sound. Obviously, they do not know the true cause of illness: immoderation. The importance of moderation led Galen, a dietetic physician, to contend that all internal diseases are caused by errors in regimen, and hence avoidable. Oswei Temkin points out that after Galen, "health ... becomes a responsibility and disease a matter for possible moral reflection" (*Galenism*, 40).

Galen's emphasis on immoderation as a cause of illness appealed to early Christians. Temkin notes, "By A.D. 350 [Galen's] acceptance as the leading authority was clearly established, and from about that time his position was secured in Alexandria, once more the center of medical learning" (*Galenism*, 61). Greco-Roman medicine held that illness was a consequence of immoderation; this view fit nicely into a Christian framework. Consequently, Greco-Roman medicine was not rejected by Christian thinkers but was Christianized.

The Christian Adoption of Medicine

Numerous historians have demonstrated how early theologians Christianized Greco-Roman medicine. Both Nancy Siraisi in *Medieval and Early Renaissance Medicine* (1990) and Carole Rawcliffe in *Medicine and Society in Later Medieval England* (1995) provide helpful and accurate introductions to the Christianization of medicine. In *Hippocrates in a World of Pagans and Christians* (1991), Oswei Temkin examines the relationship between secular and monastic medicine as Christian institutions adopted Hippocratic ideas about the body, illness, and health. Darrel Amundsen's *Medicine, Society, and Faith in the Ancient and Medieval Worlds* (1996) explores the boundaries between Christianity and medicine as drawn by both historians and medieval people. Finally, in *The Birth of the Hospital in the Byzantine Empire* (1985), Timothy Miller demonstrates how early Christians subsumed pagan sites of healing in order to replace one religion with another. By first exploring Miller's work with Christian healing places, I show how Christianity attempted to fulfill some of the social responsibilities implied by Greco-Roman belief. I then demonstrate how the boundaries between medicine and theology were relatively thin during the medieval period by examining the role of medicine in penitential literature and monastic life. While these thin boundaries existed throughout the Middle Ages, around the twelfth century medicine started to become institutionalized, and thus became more secular. But it never fully lost its connection to Christian thinking, especially the connections between illness and sin.

The Christianization of medicine is most evident in the replacement of the medical-cult god, Asklepios, with the Christian God, Jesus. Asklepios was a Greco-Roman god who passed on methods of healing and medical knowledge to his believers. According to Timothy Miller:

> When in the archaic period the god Asklepios emerged as the deity of the healing art, myth wove him into the chain of knowledge passed from generation to generation. Zeus taught Apollo; Apollo taught Asklepios; the deified Asklepios, in turn, passed the torch of medical knowledge to mortal doctors. By the fifth and fourth centuries B.C., Greek physicians regularly called themselves the Asklepiads or the Sons of Asklepios. (31)

Hippocrates considered himself one of the sons of Asklepios, and Galen believed that he was cured of an illness by Asklepios (Temkin, *Hippocrates*, 41). Whether through the passage of knowledge or through direct healing, the Greco-Roman medical system had a direct connection to the heavens. This connection played an important role in validating medicine as a divine craft.

The cult of Asklepios continued from the Greek to the Roman age. New shrines to Asklepios appeared throughout the Mediterranean (Miller 38). Archeological excavations and literary analysis provide information on how this cult worked. As Miller states,

> When a suffering person arrived in the town, he usually had to find some kind of lodging on his own. Then, he walked or was carried to the sacred shrine and entered the temple precinct. There, he made some sacrifice to Asklepios and withdrew to a section of the temple area where he could sleep. This was the famous incubation. Often the suppliant simply found a comfortable spot or brought along a mat to lay on the floor. But some temples, such as the ones at Epidauros and Phocis, maintained special buildings where the sick could sleep. While the suppliants slept, Asklepios worked his wondrous miracles in three ways. The god might simply cure the suppliant in his slumber so that he awoke in perfect health. Or, he might appear in a dream and instruct the sufferer to perform a specific action, often of a bizarre nature. Finally, he might recommend an accepted medical remedy. (40)

The cult of Asklepios continued to flourish throughout much of the fourth century. It eventually collapsed under an attack on pagan shrines by the emperor Theodosius (379–95 A.D.). Interestingly, the cult of Asklepios was not destroyed but replaced by the cults of Christian healers, the most important being Christ (Miller 33).

Early Christian writers considered medicine to be divinely sent and sanctioned.[3] Origen (185–254 A.D.) writes, "And surely there can be no doubt about medical knowledge. For if there is any knowledge [that comes] from God—which will be more so than the knowledge of health, in which the virtues of herbs as well as the qualities and differences of [the] humours are discerned?" (qtd in Temkin, *Hippocrates*, 130). Origen implies that because God has power over the natural world, the knowledge of plants and the makeup of the body's humors is divine information given to man. Therefore, medicine is divinely sent and sanctioned. As Temkin notes, "Christian theology, the biblical symbolism of disease, and biblical examples of disease of the soul transformed the pagan medicine of the soul into a spiritual medicine" (*Hippocrates* 177). Once medicine became spiritual, it was only a small move to the belief that the illnesses of the body reflected the state of the soul. But the move required the adoption of medicine under the auspices of theology.

Between the third and sixth centuries, Christianity embraced a connection between illness and sin and furthered the unity between spiritual and physical medicine. In the Old and New Testaments, disease was often a punishment to individuals who transgressed God's law; consequently, Christ becomes the physician who can cure both spiritual and physical diseases (Jeffrey 614). While Christ was thought to be the perfect physician, his followers also gained acclaim as healers and curers. David Lyle Jeffrey recognizes, "The apostle Luke, one of the four evangelists and author also of the Acts of the Apostles, is referred to by Paul as 'the beloved physician' (Col. 4:14)" (614).[4]

CHRIST, APOSTLES AND PRIESTS AS DOCTORS

The image of Christ as the perfect doctor finds a permanent place in Christian thought with the writings of Saint Ambrose (339–97 A.D.) and Saint Augustine (354–430 A.D.). According to Christian tradition, Christ was both the savior of souls and healer of bodies. In *De interpelatione Job et David*, Saint Ambrose writes that Christ "heal[s] our wounds ... He heals those that are willing and does not compel the unwilling" (qtd in Jeffrey 614). Saint Augustine also demonstrates the physical and spiritual healing of Christ. For example, in *On Christian Doctrine*, Augustine states:

> But you, O Lord, abide forever, and you will not be angry with us forever, for you have mercy on earth and ashes, and it has been pleasing in your sight to reform my deformities. By inner goads you aroused me, so that I did not rest until you stood plain before my inner sight. By the secret hand of your Physician [Christ] my swelling wound subsided, and day by day my mind's afflicted and darkened eyes grew sounder under the healing salve of sorrow. (168)

Like the members of the Asklepios cult who received healing through dreams, Augustine believes God healed him through a vision. What the healing God does for Augustine is spiritual and not physical, but the portrayal of Christ as a physician is unmistakable. More importantly, the last sentence demonstrates the addition of Christian practice into the healing process—the need for contrition. Only sorrow for one's sins invokes the healing power of God.

The Christian Church also approved patron saints to govern medical knowledge and practice. Saints Cosmas and Damien provide the clearest connection between medicine and theology. According to tradition, both saints were well known for their medical expertise when an individual came to them with a leg so infected that "the saints had to cover their noses, for he already stank, because his bone too was festering" (Temkin, *Hippocrates*, 166). The two saints attempted to turn the sufferer away, but through his insistence, they accepted him into their homes. That night, angel Raphael came to the saints and told of a dead man "whose right lower leg they should give to the wounded man." (Temkin, *Hippocrates*, 166). The saints did as the angel told them, and the man was cured. According to Temkin, the hagiography of Cosmas and Damien "explain[s] the appellation of 'anargyroi' (literally, 'without money'). The anargyroi were physician-saints who cured without any remuneration" (*Hippocrates* 166). The legend also demonstrates that the Church controlled medical knowledge, and it was sent down willingly from God.

Cosmas and Damien also demonstrate the unification of disease and sin and the importance of contrition for the alleviation of sin. Saints Cosmas and Damien's day of remembrance is 27 September, and the prayer for the patron saints reinforces that the sins of the soul are found in the infirmities of the body. The prayer states, "May this bodily infirmity be to them a spiritual medicine of the soul. What previously in health they did amiss now let them repent in their sickness. Help them after their present infirmities to deserve to possess heavenly consolations" (Beck xiii). The presence of disease suggests a period of moral reflection as the individual finds the reason for the sickness of the soul as refracted through the body. During the first six centuries of the common era, Christianity adopted pagan beliefs about disease and health and Christianized them by creating a spiritual medicine. With this theory firmly in place, all medical learning was framed by Christian thought.

Once the Church sanctioned medicine, the priest could also be a physician. As Carole Rawcliffe states, "The idea of *Christus Medicus* (Christ as doctor/healer) derived from the writings of St. Augustine of Hippo (d. 430), where Christ's ordeal on the cross is compared to the act of a devoted physician who reassures his patient by tasting unpleasant medicine first" (*Source* 4). In *On Christian Doctrine* (c. 396), Augustine develops the idea that the crucifixion of Christ is a cure for sickness as well as sin: "Just as a cure is the way to health, so also this Cure received sinners to heal and strengthen them" (14). Christ attends to the sinner's wounds as would a doctor, by sometimes applying similar or contrary elements: "He who tends the wounds of the body sometimes applies contraries, such as cold to hot, moist to dry, and so on; at other times he applies similar things" (Augustine 15). Augustine points out that because man fell through the sin of Pride, God acted like a doctor when he applied the contrary, Humility, as the cure. This is also true when Christ's virtues cure man's vices. But God also cures, like a doctor, by using similar elements, such as when a woman, Eve, deceived man, God used another woman, Mary, to free man, and when God used the death of His Son to free man from spiritual death. Augustine concludes, "the Wisdom of God, setting out to cure men, applied Himself to cure them, being once the Physician and the Medicine" (15). Once God and Christ are structured as the physicians who heal human souls, it is not much of a leap to the belief that the priest would also have access to both spiritual and physical medicines.

After Greek medicine was Christianized, Christian authors relied heavily on the relationship between spiritual and bodily illness. Because of Galen's association of immoderation with illness and because of medicine's growing part in Christian theology, medieval medical doctors developed theories that argued that some illnesses reflected immoral states. Thus, some illnesses both result from sins committed against God and require moral reflection and contrition. Through an examination of the sins that medieval people connected to disease, I am able to show not only that these moral associations were literal, but also that these associations reflect social concerns of the medieval period. In other words, when medieval people stated that envy caused leprosy, they meant that this sin literally caused leprosy. A person who is envious can threaten the stability and health of the community; therefore, God identifies him or her as a threat through the sign of the disease, and it is the people's responsibility to recognize the sign, interpret the sign, and remove the person from the community. Medicine gives rise to a philosophy that examines both the individual and the individual's relationship to the community.

Medicine as Part of Natural Philosophy

The belief that medicine was a component of philosophy was so thoroughly ingrained in the thought of Christian authors that it became a common way to approach spiritual sickness. The relationship between medicine and philosophy is most evident in Boethius's *The Consolation of Philosophy* (c. 524). Here Philosophy uses medicine as an analogy to explain the nature of a healthy soul:

> For it is a mystery to the layman why some healthy persons find sweet foods agreeable, others sour foods, and why some sick persons are helped by gentle treatment, others by harsh medicines. The physician, however, does not find such things at all strange because he understands the nature of sickness and health. Now, what is the health of souls but virtue, and what is their sickness but vice? And who, indeed, is the preserver of the good and the corrector of the wicked but God, the governor and physician of men's minds, who looks into the great mirror of his providence and, knowing what is best for each one, causes it to happen? Here, then, is the great miracle of the order of Fate: divine wisdom does what the ignorant cannot understand. (94)

According to Philosophy, illness is related both literally and metaphorically to the health of the soul. As Philosophy states, God is the governor and physician of men's minds and the corrector of the wicked. Therefore, by indirection, illness results both from men's sins and from God's attempt to provide correction.

Each illness requires a period of moral reflection during which the individual can interpret the meaning of the disease. By correcting one's mind, Philosophy can also correct one's health. This is evident when Dame Philosophy rebukes the Muses of Poetry:

> Who let these whores from the theater come to the bedside of this sick man? They cannot offer medicine for his sorrows, they will nourish him only with their sweet poison. They kill the fruitful harvest of reason with the sterile thorns of the passions; they do not liberate the minds of men from disease, but merely accustom them to it. I would find it easier to bear if your flattery had, as it usually does, seduced some ordinary dull-witted man; in that case, it would have been no concern of mine. But this man has been educated in the philosophical schools of the Eleatics and the Academy. Get out, you Sirens; your sweetness leads to death. Leave him to be cured and made strong by my Muses. (4–5).

For Boethius, poetry can only resign people to disease. Philosophy, on the other hand, can cure all disease, for Philosophy can free man from the shackles of mortal thoughts. As Dame Philosophy states, " 'But it is time for medicine rather than complaint ... To bring you to your senses, I shall quickly wipe the dark cloud of mortal things from your eyes.' Then, she dried my tear-filled eyes with a fold of her robe" (6). This statement rephrases Augustine's claim that God visits man and heals his eyes through sorrow. By wiping Boethius's eyes, Philosophy cures his blindness. One aspect of Boethius's blindness is that he fails to remember that illness is the consequence of immorality.

The connection between medicine and theology was not confined to the Church fathers. Religious institutions were also involved in the study and transmission of medical ideas. From the seventh through the twelfth century, the monastery was the seat of medical learning for the community, because secular medical education at a university was not available until the twelfth century—for example, at Paris and Salerno (Siraisi, *Medieval*, 48). Siraisi declares:

> As time went by, the medical knowledge and healing activity tended to come more and more within the orbit of ecclesiastical communities. To the extent that it involved book learning and the transmission of Greco-Roman doctrine, medicine, like other learned disciplines, survived in western Europe between the seventh or eighth and the eleventh centuries mainly in a clerical or monastic environment. However, monks did not copy or read medical books merely as an academic exercise; Cassiodorus, in an influential work on studies appropriate for monks, recommended books by Hippocrates, Galen, and Dioscorides while linking the purpose of medical reading with charity, care, and help. (*Medieval* 10)

At Oxford and Cambridge, medical training most likely was in place by the thirteenth century, but this training was a minor course of study, usually connected to Philosophy.[5] The first medical university in England was established in 1423, then disbanded and reestablished in 1518 (Beck 62 and Siraisi, *Medieval*, 18). Prior to the twelfth century, most medical learning occurred in monasteries. The study of medicine became an important theological component for two primary reasons. First, medicine, as structured by Greco-Roman thought, could be easily Christianized, thereby layering sin on top of *sophrosyne*. Second, since no secular institution was responsible for training and making available medical practitioners, the Church became the organization by which medical aid was administered to the community.

The Monastic Transmission and Use of Medicine

The belief that illness was the result of immorality, the influence theology had on medicine, and the role priests played in helping the sick can be clearly illustrated through the penitential literature of the seventh through twelfth centuries. In *The Literature of Penance in Anglo Saxon England*, Allen J. Frantzen writes, "Penance was not a punishment: it was a cure. And the penitential was not only a list of sins and penalties for them; it was a blueprint for the sinner's conversion, didactic or catechetical as well as disciplinary" (4). The role of the penitential was to provide a better life for the penitent, both spiritually and physically, and the authors of the penitentials were not alone in attempting to improve the lives of Christians. Frantzen believes:

> Much medieval literature seeks to guide its audience along this path, but only certain texts do so with explicit references to confession and penance, and these materials—homilies and prayers and poems—join with the handbooks to constitute "penitential literature." They are "penitential" to the degree that they depend, for form or theme, on confession and acts of penance as described in the handbook. (12)

The confession is a way of reflecting on and ruminating about one's life. Penance is what one pays for an immoderate life. Health and illness relate to the penitential handbooks because the state of the soul is reflected in the body. Illness demands interpretation, and health becomes an individual's responsibility. Frantzen sees a similar responsibility in the handbooks as a whole: "Collectively, [penitential handbooks] amplified the penitential's emphasis on the individual and his need to assume responsibility for his spiritual welfare" (13). Galen created a medical philosophy in which health was the responsibility of each individual, and the penitentials proposed a spiritual health also dependent on individual will. It should be of no surprise then that the penitential handbooks blurred boundaries between the discourses of medicine and theology, between the body and the soul, since the body reflected the soul's health.

The most influential work on medicine in the penitentials is John T. McNeill's "Medicine for Sin as Prescribed in the Penitentials"; however, McNeill's work is compromised by his assumption that the penitentials relied on Methodist ideology rather than Galenic. McNeill attempts to investigate why the "penitent was regarded as one morally diseased and ill, and his treatment is, in the Penitentials, repeatedly, even habitually, referred to as the task of the moral physician. His sins are the symptoms of disease" ("Medicine," 14). Within the penitential literature, one sees the growth of spiritual medicine in which the state of the soul is reflected on the body. McNeill argues that the penitentials are influenced by the Methodist sect's medical notion of tense and relaxed. As McNeill states, "Historians are of the opinion that Soranus, with his emphasis on the contraries and his special attention to obstetrics, was much better known than Galen, whose contributions to physiology and anatomy were not greatly appreciated by his contemporaries" ("Medicine,"16). While this may have been true when McNeill was writing in 1926, much has changed in the study of the history of medicine.

As Siraisi demonstrates, both Galen and Hippocrates were well known by Cassiodorus, but Soranus, a Greek physician and author from the first century A.D., is not mentioned. Furthermore, in both *Galenism: Rise and Decline of a Medical Philosophy* and *Hippocrates in a World of Pagans and Christians*, Temkin argues conclusively that Hippocrates and Galen were the leading medical authorities throughout the Middle Ages and Early Modern Period. Therefore, the penitential's reference to contraries most likely refers to the idea of humoral contraries as developed by Hippocrates and Galen, rather than to body-surface contraries of tense and relaxed as argued by the Methodists via Soranus. While McNeill understandably errs in his claim that the penitentials are informed by Methodist medical thought, he is correct in believing that Greco-Roman medicine was Christianized in the Penitentials and that the sins of the soul are reflected in the body.

Numerous penitential works use medical language, primarily references to contraries, to explain the nature of sin and the role of the confessor. The Penitential of Columban (c.600) states:

> The talkative person is to be sentenced to silence, the disturber to gentleness, the gluttonous to fasting, the sleepy fellow to watchfulness, the proud to imprisonment, the deserter to expulsion. Diversity of guilt occasions diversity of penalty; for even the physicians of bodies prepare their remedies in various sorts. For they treat wounds in one way, fevers, in another, burns in another. So therefore the spiritual physicians ought to heal with various sorts of treatment the wounds, fevers, transgressions, sorrows, sicknesses, and infirmities of souls. (qtd in McNeill, "Medicine," 18)

Both the priest and doctor cure by using the opposite or contrary to establish a balance. The balance that the spiritual doctor is trying to achieve is not that different from the one Galen attempted in his medical work.

Medicine and theology, doctor and priest, are unified through the idea that each day's events have the potential to damage one's physical or spiritual health. Just as physical metaphors are used in the penitentials, spiritual metaphors are used in the medical works. In his discussion about the unification of philosophy and medicine through Galen and Hippocrates, Temkin states:

> The philosopher's concern was with the soul and its aspiration to knowledge, virtue, and beauty. Vices, including uncontrolled passion, crime against man, and sin against the gods, were diseases of the soul, which the philosopher had to cure. The doctor's primary concern with the soul was with the diseases from which it suffered concomitantly with the body as well as with the reactions its perturbances provoked in the body. Galen mentioned 'passion, weeping, anger, grief, immoderate worry, and much sleeplessness' as bringing on 'fevers and the beginnings of severe diseases . . . just as, on the other hand, a sluggish mind and mindlessness, and an altogether spiritless soul often produce lack of color and atrophies.' Whatever their individual explanations were, most authors of the Collection would probably have accepted this interrelationship of body and soul. The two were not felt to be separated by as deep a gulf as Descartes later envisioned. (*Hippocrates*, 14)

The unity between the body and the soul, between philosophy and medicine, and between illness and sin plays a large part in how priests in the penitential manuals see their social function. For example, *The Penitential of Theodore*, written by Theodore of Tarsus, Archbishop of Canterbury (668–690 A.D.) demonstrates the connection between priest and physician. In the Preface to the penitential, the author describes Theodore as one of the "physicians to the souls" (McNeill, *Penance,* 182). This tag demonstrates medicine's metaphoric placement within religion. The role of the priest is to cure the soul just as the role of a physician is to cure the body.

The early penitentials sought to provide a balance to life much like the Galenic doctors of the Greco-Roman period. As McNeill states, "in large degree the Penitentials seek to recover to the offender a balanced state of mind. There is nothing that impresses itself more upon the student of the Penitentials than their moderation, fundamental humaneness and freedom from fanaticism" ("Medicine," 20). What we see in the penitentials is Greco-Roman medicine modified to fit a Christian structure. Temkin states, "What was to distinguish the sincere Christian doctor from a pagan was a new relationship to his faith and its church rather than a fundamental change in his professional ethics" (*Hippocrates* 35). From the sixth to twelfth centuries, a priest would be a doctor to soul, but the soul was also believed to influence the health of the body. Therefore, a priest becomes a physician both to the soul and body because medicine was part of natural philosophy and because monasteries housed most of the medical knowledge during this period. The organization that houses medical manuscripts has governance of medical learning. The Church's influence on medicine would provide the foundation for a moral interpretation of disease.

Moral interpretations of diseases reflect common social fears of a period. These interpretations are not haphazard, but rather intentional. Moreover, they are designed to improve society by demonstrating that certain moral failings receive physical punishments. The uninfected are supposed to learn from the infected and, thus, avoid the sin that led to the illness. As McNeill states, "We have no means of knowing how often the more heinous offences noted in the Penitentials were actually committed; but we may be sure that the saintly men who wrote these books did not invent merely hypothetical sins. They were dealing with real life as they themselves had closely observed it" ("Medicine," 21–22). Both the role of medicine and the connections between sin and illness in the penitentials highlight social problems people faced in the early Middle Ages. Few people had access to learned medicine, so the penitentials helped to provide access to it through a priest's dissemination of medical information in the confessional. Further, the connection between certain sins and illnesses in the penitentials illustrates social fears common to those people and that period.

While it is possible to argue that a medical connection in the penitential manuals is merely metaphoric, it is hard to dispute the purpose of certain lines of information that clearly point literally to medicine, especially in the category "Of the Use or Rejection of Animals" in *The Penitential of Theodore*. In this category, the author declares, "The hare may be eaten, and it is good for dysentery; and its gall is to be mixed with pepper for the [relief of] pain" (McNeill, *Penance*, 208). When one considers all the potential reasons for dysentery during the Middle Ages, from unsanitary sewer systems to spoiled food, this ailment would most likely be epidemic. In reference to specific water-borne diseases, Robert Gottfried writes, "The deadliest [illnesses] were infantile diarrhea, dehydration from which was a major cause of infant mortality, as high as 50 percent of all children, and intestinal dysentery, the 'bloody flux' " (*Black Death*, 134). Likewise, the number of people who would be suffering from pain would also be substantial. Therefore, it would be logical to provide priests with information on an apparent cure for or relief from dysentery. Few people would have had access to trained medical doctors.

Penitential literature also evinces fears concerning common medical practices of pagan origin. Again in *Theodore*, under the category "Of the worship of Idols," the author writes, "If any woman puts her daughter upon a roof or into an oven for the cure of a fever, she shall do penance for seven years" (McNeill, *Penance*, 198). Amundsen explains injunctions against pagan rites in Christian Penitentials: "The placing of a child upon a roof or into (or on) an oven for the cure of a fever was frequently condemned. The oven (or hearth) was the place where the guardian spirits of the house dwelt; spirits who might aid healing also resided on the roof" (185). The inclusion of these pagan beliefs point to an important social relationship: medicine, both folk and academic, and theology were interrelated. Frantzen states:

> The confessor was also a teacher, and the confessional encounter, more than simply a judgment of the sinner, was an opportunity for correction and instruction ... [T]he priest's role as confessor was linked to his duties as a teacher and, in all probability, a preacher. All his pastoral skills converged in confession, and his guide in exercising them was the penitential. (10)

Through the confessional, the priest could have instructed the penitent in academic medicine and restricted the use of pagan folklore. Medicine and theology did not stand in contrast to each other; rather each discipline informed the other and influenced how people of the Middle Ages lived.

Many of the penitentials focus on the collection of herbs, an activity that is important to both paganism and medicine. It is easy to see how Christian writers needed to keep a collection of herbs for medical purposes but attempted to regulate the activity within a Christian framework. In *Theodore*, under "Of Those Who Are Vexed by the Devil," the author writes, "One who is possessed of a demon may have stones and herbs, without [the use of] incantations" (McNeill, *Penance*, 207). In *The Penitential of Silos* (ca. 800), the author writes, "It is not permitted to observe [the customs connected with] wool at the Kalends, or the collections of herbs, [or] to give heed to incantations except to perform everything with the creed and the Lord's prayer" (McNeill, *Penance*, 288). The same information is included in *The Corrector and Physician* of Burchard of Worms (ca.1008–12), Chapter 65 (Amundsen 185). Amundsen concludes that in penitential literature that mentions healing, "[t]here is no indication that the sickness was regarded as a punishment for sin, because the penitent was to resume penance if he or she recovered from his or her illness. Nothing here was even implied about causality" (185). While it is true that there seems to be little direct causality between illness and sin in the penitentials, it is hard to ignore that certain medical procedures, such as herb collection and incantation, had sinful possibilities. More importantly, confession follows medical practices in having the penitent / patient reflects on his or her sinful nature. If the body mirrors the state of the soul, the act of confession would bring health to both the soul and the body.

The theology of medicine is especially clear in monastic communities, many of which were the repository of medical texts and knowledge. Bede (672–735) demonstrates some of the earliest beliefs about medicine's role in monastic life. In Bede's *Life of St Cuthbert* (c.721), Cuthbert (c.634–687) has a disfiguring facial disease: "when he lived a communal life among the brethren, the symptoms of this illness were clearly seen upon his face" (Colgrave 305).[6] Cuthbert is asked by "many devout persons ... to give them some portion of the relics" (Colgrave 305).[7] Cuthbert decides to give them a piece of the skin of a calf that he has used to block the wind and rain, but prior to giving them the calf skin, Cuthbert uses a piece of it for himself. Bede writes, "[H]e put a part of the same skin into water and washed his face with it, and immediately all the swelling which had covered it and the loathsome scab departed"(Colgrave 305).[8] This tale demonstrates the power of the monastic community to relieve illnesses much as a doctor would with a salve. Bede interprets Cuthbert's treatment to "the grace of Almighty God, who, in this present age, is wont to heal many, and, in time to come, will heal our diseases of mind and body" (Colgrave 307).[9] While Bede ascribes the cure to divine intervention, he also supports the use of salves, at least in this case, that alleviate physical pain. Cuthbert is not meant to live in physical pain. Rather because of his devote and pious ways, Cuthbert is shown by God how to cure his physical ailment.

Since most medical manuscripts were kept and copied in monasteries, the monastic community not only had access to this information, but also controlled medical discourse. Monastic orders became the most knowledgeable medical practitioners from the seventh to the twelfth centuries. The Benedictine order, more than any other order, is known for its involvement in medicine. As Temkin notes,

> Saint Benedict's rule made the care of the sick brethren a prime obligation 'before and above' all others. The abbot had to see to it that they were not neglected, while they, on their side, had to keep in mind that they were servants of God and were obligated not to sadden the brethren serving them by making excessive demands. No mention was made of physicians; but if inference from Cassiodorus is permissible, monks with some medical knowledge would have been chosen to look after the sick. (*Hippocrates* 155)

Other monastic orders did not place similar importance on caring for health. The Cistercians of the eleventh century seem, at least upon first reading, to oppose medical learning because they refused to partake in it. However, David N. Bell refutes the idea that Cistercians were opposed to medical intercession or knowledge. Bell identifies the passage of Saint Bernard of Clairvaux (1090–1154) that has led most scholars to believe that Cistercians condemned medicine: "Puta te, quaeso, monachum esse, non medicum, nec de complexione iudicandum, sed de professione" (qtd. in Bell 140). Scholars focus on Bernard's claim that Cistercians are not physicians, "medicum," but monks, "monachum." This passage, however, demonstrates that medicine was taught in all monasteries, perhaps to such a degree that Bernard believed the monks were more concerned with bodily rather than spiritual salvation.

To further his argument that Cistercians did not ban medicine within the monastery, Bell examines the records of practicing doctors, the medical manuscripts housed in the monasteries, and the hospitals associated with the order. Bell argues that other scholars believe, "Every large Benedictine monastery in the twelfth and thirteenth centuries (says Hammond) could boast a trained or self-taught physician; but, says he, 'I venture no such conjecture . . . for the Cluniacs, Cistercians, and Carthusians, whose service to England was generally without distinction and whose chronicles are few' " (150). In opposition to these statements, Bell uses Talbot and Hammond's compilation of medical practitioners in medieval England and finds fourteen physicians that attended the Cistercian sick. Added to this, Bell finds three more that are identified by Kealey in *Medieval Medicus* (150). Bell writes, "Eleven of the *medici* appear to date from the second half of the twelfth century, and six from the first half of the thirteenth century. After that they seem to fade away" (151). While doctors serving the monastery are not monks, this implies that Cistercians did partake of medical practice and had at least some access to medical professionals and services. Unlike the Benedictines who practiced medicine within the monastery, the Cistercians practiced disciplinary boundaries between medicine and theology by inviting doctors in only when necessary.

Even though the Cistercians were attempting to separate medical from theological practice, Cistercian abbeys still housed medical manuscripts that would have been available to the monks, as Bell shows. While far from impressive, the numbers are comparable to those in monasteries of other orders (159). Bell writes, "All that we can conclude from the list of medical texts in Cistercian libraries is that such treatises were certainly there; but we cannot conclude that what is recorded necessarily represents the sum total" (160). What the list does represent is that *pharmacopoeia* was important to monasteries and "every monastery would have had a herb–garden" (Bell 160). Bell concludes, "Cistercian libraries certainly contained medical treatises, both classical and contemporary, and under no circumstances must it be suggested that the comparative paucity of the evidence reflects a corresponding disinterest in the topic" (172). Even within Cistercian orders, medicine seems to have been studied and practiced by members of the monastery.

Cistercians also created numerous infirmaries throughout England. Bell finds twenty-six places where medical care could have been given to the laity (171). Many of these infirmaries were established in the early thirteenth century and some functioned to various degrees as leprosariums and almshouses. As Bell concludes about these infirmaries:

> The spaciousness and richness of many of the thirteenth-century infirmaries, together with the obvious importance of the infirmarer with his separate lodgings, indicate that at this period the monastic hospital was in no way a secondary or subordinate structure ... the documentary evidence of some twenty-six hospitals and hospices associated with the Order leads one to suspect that the Cistercians were more deeply concerned about the local population than one might suspect (172).

From Bell's study, it is evident that even the Order, which historians have assumed to be the least involved with medicine, is still highly involved, although a movement toward disciplinary boundaries can be seen. The

Church's involvement with medicine shaped the approaches people took toward illness. Even when medicine became more secularized in the thirteenth and fourteenth centuries, doctors still approached disease from a Christian moral perspective.

The Secularization of Medicine

By the thirteenth century, medicine seems to have become more institutionalized and to have moved partially outside the aegis of theology. In *The Cutting Edge*, Theodore Beck lists the restrictions placed on priest-physicians in the early part of the twelfth century:

> The Council of Rheims (A.D. 1131) being the first and least severe in that whilst it prevented priests and monks from being present at public lectures on medicine it still permitted private study. By the Council of Tours (A.D. 1163) Pope Alexander III forbade the clergy to undertake surgery and this enactment finally terminated in that Canon of the Fourth Lateran Council (A.D. 1215) which ordered all subdeacons, deacons, and priests to abstain from the practice of surgery, particularly that which involved burning or cutting (all external conditions such as skin diseases and ulcers came within the province of surgery), under penalty of excommunication. Pope Honorius III (A.D. 1216–1227) extended the prohibition to the practice of medicine. (7)

The reason surgery was prohibited is that blood was considered unclean, and clergy were to avoid all uncleanness. It would appear that this prohibition was not always followed, because three well-known surgical practitioners, Lanfrank of Milan, Henri de Mondeville, and Guy de Chauliac, all took holy orders and continued to practice medicine and surgery (O'Boyle 162). Furthermore, the lower orders were still allowed to practice healing (Beck 7). What changed was the institutional nature of medicine within theology. No longer were the monasteries the storehouses of medical knowledge. Instead the university was developing. The growing institutional boundaries between medicine and theology can be seen primarily in the penitential literature of the thirteenth century.

While penitential literature prior to the thirteenth century offered priests certain amounts of medical knowledge, the penitentials after the thirteenth century lack such overt medical references. Chaucer's *The Parson's Tale*, for example, is a penitential treatise that combines three medieval works on penance and sin. Helen Cooper explains,

> His material on the nature of penitence, contrition, the conditions of confession, and satisfaction (80–386, 958–1080) is adapted from the *Summa de poenitentia* of the Dominican Raymund of Pennaforte, written in the 1220s. The account of the sins (390–955) is ultimately derived from an ency-

> clopaedia of the vices, the *Summa vitiorum*, written by another Dominican, William Peraldus, in 1236.... Chaucer also used the *Summa virtutum de remediis anime*, a work on the remedial virtues, that is, that correct the sins: humility against pride and so on. (400–1)

All three works were written after the Fourth Lateran Council ruling of 1215, and nowhere within Chaucer's penitentials do we see the recipes for dysentery or pain that were common in the earlier penitentials. Furthermore, one no longer sees the admonitions against pagan rites for curing fevers and against herbal collections that were also common to earlier penitentials.

This is not to say that Chaucer's work is completely devoid of medical reference; it just lacks the practical medical remedies seen in earlier penitentials. Chaucer's Parson still mentions the medical idea of moderation in eating: "at every tyme that a man eteth or drynketh moore than suffiseth to the sustenaunce of his body, in certein he dooth synne" (X.372). And later: "and somtyme the richesse of a man is cause of his deth; somtyme the delices of a man bese cause of the grevous maladye thurgh which he dyeth" (X.471). Instead of specific ailments and methods of curing those ailments, the later penitentials deal in general states of health. There is not a specific ailment like dysentery, but general references to maladies. The only somewhat specific reference to a medical condition occurs in relation to abortion: "whan man destroubeth concepcioun of a child, and maketh a womman outher bareyne by drynkynge venenouse herbes thurgh which she may nat conceyve, or sleeth a child by drynkes wilfully, or elles putteth certeine material thynges in hire secree places to slee the child" they shall be guilty of homicide (X.575). This reference is simply a prohibition against abortion, not a recipe to help people in times of illness. The prohibition also lacks specificity; it does not state what type of herbs, drinks, or material things that could cause an abortion primarily because that information could potentially train people to perform the abortions that the Church is trying to prohibit. These penitentials are not interested in transmitting medical knowledge to a larger audience; instead, the penitentials indicate social problems that community authorities want controlled. The lack of any overt medical references in the later penitentials points to the increasing secularization of medicine. Siraisi writes,

> The oldest universities, in France, England, Italy, and the Iberian peninsula, appeared in the late twelfth and thirteenth centuries. Although their development was legitimated, regulated, and encouraged by religious and local and regional political authorities, almost all of them came into being more or less spontaneously, and their origins involved some degree of autonomous self-assertion by scholars or masters. (*Medieval* 47)

The autonomous self-assertion enabled medicine to move from the control of religious authorities to that of the secular authorities. No longer are monks the sole repository of medical knowledge. Evidently, by the twelfth and thirteenth centuries, secular doctors are becoming more available to the general public. However, the increase of secular doctors may also increase the number of abortions performed in the community. As John Riddle has demonstrated, abortives were common in the twelfth century (118–126). The penitentials seem to reflect both the institutionalization and secularization of medicine and the social problems that these developments then cause.

While there is little reference to specific medical cures in the later penitentials, the connection between medicine and theology, or more specifically disease and sin, was by this time firmly established. Theology provided the filter through which all other events, including bodily events, could be viewed. For example, in the discussion on Luxury, the Parson declares that it occurs "[s]omtyme of langwissynge of body, for the humours been to ranke and to habundaunt in the body of man; somtyme of infermetee, for the fieblesse of the vertu retentif, as phisik maketh mencion" (X.912). The Parson illustrates the belief that certain sins are reflected in the ailments of the body. At times, the body and the body's humors allow one to slip into the sin of luxury. The remedy is common contrary therapy: the penitent is to practice chastity and continence.

Medicine's involvement with theology shaped the way medieval people looked at disease. The early Church altered the Greco-Roman belief that medicine was part of natural philosophy and spiritualized medicine. Christ and his followers became doctors who were entrusted with the well being both of the bodies and souls they served. Disease and health were Christianized so that the body reflected the state of the soul. Christian doctors were not the first to interpret disease through a moral framework. Rather, they moved the moral interpretation of disease and health into the metaphysical realm of sin, punishment, and redemption.

Obviously not every illness encountered by medieval people was connected to a moral failing. Some illnesses were believed to occur naturally or as a result of old age. Amundsen's caution concerning modern interpretations of medieval beliefs is worth quoting at length:

> Another commonplace encountered in modern assessments of the early Middle Ages is the assertion that early medieval people saw sin as the cause of most sickness. Here there is room for much confusion because the relationship of sin with sickness can appear at three different levels. First, sin was certainly regarded by early medieval authors as the cause of sickness in the sense that without sin there would have been no material evil. This, although not expressed, was an underlying assumption of the sources. Second, one's own general sinfulness was often given as the cause of one's own sickness. Third, sickness, it was thought, might result from a specific sin. This last statement is very seldom encountered except in denunciations of and warnings to entire communities, and then the emphasis was often on general moral laxity, which makes it nearly indistinguishable from the

> second category. We should also note that it is one thing to maintain that a person is sick as a punishment for a specific sin to which he or she is obstinately and tenaciously clinging, but it is quite another matter to attribute one's own sickness to one's general sinfulness and see the sickness as part of God's punitive and refining process. (187–8)

Dysentery or gum disease certainly would have unclear moral connections because these diseases affected everybody, but leprosy and bubonic plague are two diseases that clearly fit Amundsen's categories. Amundsen rightly recognizes this when he writes,

> Sin was commonly regarded as the immediate cause of plague, or at least the catalyst behind God's sending the plague. This was collective sin. Individual sin was seldom seen as the cause of sickness, whether mental illness or physical ailments. One notable exception was leprosy, which was associated with a variety of sins, but especially with lust and pride (210).

Amundsen correctly notes that leprosy and bubonic plague were associated with individual and collective sins, respectively. However, a detailed study of the variety of sins associated with leprosy will demonstrate that leprosy was not connected with lust as the primary moral cause of the disease. The moral associations of certain diseases in the medieval period are important both to the accurate understanding of certain literary works that employ these diseases as a method of character development and to the perceived ills of the society.

Leprosy and bubonic plague are combined through the role Christianity played in the interpretation and construction of each disease. Leprosy afflicts an individual and therefore can be dealt with privately as each case erupts. The leper is the other who has personally sinned against God. In response, God has sent the leper this disease which signifies the leper's sin and identifies him as a moral and social threat. During the Middle Ages, leprosy represented spiritual sins, particularly pride, envy, avarice or anger. Leprosy gained new venereal associations with the advent of syphilis in the Renaissance. Leprosy, like syphilis, is individuated because the individual leper is justly punished for his or her sin. Moreover, the construction of the disease fits nicely into human dichotomies of the healthy and the ill. The leper shows outward signs of the disease which enables others to identify him as part of the kingdom of the ill.

Bubonic plague seems to have prompted a different response than leprosy. In this case, an individuated response did not exist; rather, the epidemic nature of the disease left both sinner and saint punished. Bubonic plague was seen as a sign of a massive moral failing, a common breaking of the covenant with God, and a collective punishment. Control of this disease by individual Christian practice was impossible because it affected everyone. Moreover, bubonic plague is an acute disease in which sufferers either die or recover in a short period of time. There was little need to establish long-term care as was done for lepers. Therefore, the comfortable dichotomy of healthy and ill was not as easily established since the disease attacked so quickly.

Contemporary society still retains many of the medieval connections between illness and morality, connections that influence literature as well as society. The clearest literary example of both the influence of medicine on literature and the connection between morality and illness appears in our own adjectives: sanguine, choleric, phlegmatic, and melancholy. At one time, these adjectives referred to the emotional and moral state of the individual as well as to his or her physical constitution. More importantly, these adjectives are used throughout the literature of the Middle Ages, but few critics have examined them in a literal way. For example, in the Middle English lyric, "Thirty Dayes Hath November," the author sums up the moral and physical associations:

Fleumaticus:
Sluggy and slowe, in spetinge muiche,
Cold and moist, my natur is suche;
Dull of wit, and fat, of contenaunce strange,
Fleumatike, this complecion may not change.

Sanguineus:
Deliberal I am, loving and gladde,
Laghinge and playing, full seld I am sad;
Singing, full fair of colour, bold to fight,
Hote and moist, beninge, sanguine I hight.

Colericus:
I am sad and soleynge with heviness in thoght;
I covet right muiche, leve will I noght;
Fraudulent and suttill, full cold and dry,
Yollowe of colour, colorike am I.

Malencolicus:
Envius, dissevabill, my skin is roghe;
Outrage in exspence, hardy inoghe,
Suttill and sklender, hote and dry,
Of colour pale, my nam is malencoly. (Luria 112)

Each one of these dominant humors corresponds to an emotional state which, if indulged to excess, could lend itself to sin. The assumptions which underlie this poem are that being phlegmatic may lead to the sin of idleness, being sanguine may lead to the sins of lust and overindulgence, being choleric may lead to the sin of covetousness, and being melancholic may lead to the sins of deceit and envy. When a medieval author used these adjectives to describe literary characters, the medieval reader would have easily connected the adjective to its equivalent sin. Not only were humors connected to sins, but so were certain diseases, such as leprosy and bubonic plague. Around each of these diseases lies a discourse in which the medical, theological, and literary disciplines influenced the interpretation of the disease.

There is still much work to be done in relation to medieval medicine and its connection to social groups. This book attempts to fill a void in one aspect of this scholarship. By examining the connection between morality and illness, I seek to demonstrate an interaction among medicine, theology, and literature which has not been examined. This interaction points to the need to take medieval authors' connection between morality and disease on a literal, rather than a metaphoric level, because both doctors and priests believed that immorality led to illnesses.

For too long critics have maintained disciplinary boundaries which were not part of the medieval system. Evidence for the close relation between medicine and theology comes directly from a Chaucerian passage. In the *Physician's Tale*, the Physician states that Envy is sorry for other men's well-being and is glad for other's sorrow and misery (115–6). The Physician then states: "The Doctour maketh this descripcioun" (117). Next to this passage in the Hengrwrt and Ellesmere manuscripts the scribes wrote the Latin gloss "Augustinus" (Skeat 263 n.117). The relation between medicine and theology is so close in the Middle Ages that some scribe apparently needed to mark the text so as not to create a misreading of who the physician's "Doctour" is. Furthermore, the lines the Physician quotes from Augustine are then quoted in a longer form by another religious figure—the Parson (X. 484). What is evident from this quotation is that medicine is informed by theology, and this information finds its way into the literature of the period.

The only way to understand the role of disease in literature from other time periods is first to examine how different social groups interpreted the disease. It is then possible to see how literary authors use these diseases to inform their characters and plot. The next chapter examines the construction and interpretation of leprosy, bubonic plague, and syphilis as medicine and theology inform them.

CHAPTER TWO

Leprosy, Bubonic Plague, and Syphilis

This chapter provides a historical overview of leprosy, bubonic plague, and syphilis in the Middle Ages and Renaissance and a history of the scholarship surrounding each disease. Essentially, I examine the early moral associations of each disease and how those associations changed over time. For the purposes of this chapter, I am looking at how medical and theological communities participated and interacted in the construction of the reception of disease. As I demonstrated in the last chapter, medicine was increasingly moving towards secularization, but it was not entirely free from the effects of theology, especially in relation to interpretation. Consequently, both medical and theological communities interpreted these three diseases through a moral filter that saw disease as a divine punishment sent to correct man's sins. This chapter explains the foundation through which the medical and theological communities interpreted disease. With this foundation in place, I am able to examine the cultural meaning of disease as implied by literary authors who participated in and transmitted these ideas to a larger social body.

Leprosy and the Seven Deadly Sins

No disease exemplifies Susan Sontag's passport metaphor better than leprosy. Unlike other diseases in which the sick remained with the healthy, leprosy truly gave one access to a new domain, the kingdom of the lepers. In 1179, the Third Lateran Council suggested that a ceremony take place in which the leper was pronounced dead to the world and separated from "the company of persons." The ceremony differed from place to place. England was the most lax in sequestration; however, the ceremony had some consistent outlines.[1] Priests, and in some locations medical doctors, would investigate reports and diagnose leprosy. Once the officials believed that leprosy was present on the victim, the victim was removed from his or her house and brought to a ceremonial location, either a church or a graveyard. The ceremony was very similar to a burial ceremony: the leper was pronounced dead to the world. In some cases, the leper crawled into an open grave or had three shovels of dirt thrown on his or her head. After the ceremony, the leper would put on clothes befitting the leper's new social role and be given a device that he or she would use to warn of approach, usually a rattle, castanet, or bell (Brody 66). The leper would then have to move to a new location outside of town where he or she would have to live off the alms of the populace. Forced to accept a new house, new clothes, and new occupation, the leper had truly emigrated to a new kingdom.

It is widely held in the Middle Ages that leprosy was a punishment for lechery. It is my contention instead that leprosy was connected to a variety of sins including envy, wrath, and avarice, but very rarely lechery. Throughout the medieval period, the sins most commonly associated with leprosy were from the spiritual, rather than carnal categories. Morton Bloomfield argues that, from the seventh century on, most medieval people followed Gregory the Great's list of seven deadly sins in which "[t]he first five Sins are spiritual and the last two carnal" (73). The five spiritual sins are Pride, Envy, Anger, Avarice, and Sloth. The carnal sins are Lechery and Gluttony. Cassian (d. c.435) believed that the two carnal sins were natural because "[f]or the preservation of the human race we must indulge, to some extent at least, in *gula* and *fornicatio*, whereas there is no such compulsion in the case of the other five" (Bloomfield 70). During the medieval period there was a greater emphasis on the spiritual sins than carnal, and the sins that were associated with leprosy often come from the spiritual categories, not the carnal.

Other diseases, such as bubonic plague and syphilis, were also originally connected to the spiritual sins, but eventually were altered, especially in the case of syphilis, to include the carnal sins. This movement from spiritual to carnal sins demonstrates an attempt to harness disease under human control, since carnality is easier to control than pride. However, most scholars want to connect leprosy in the Middle Ages to the sins of carnality, rather than to those of spirituality, even though most of the textual evidence points to the latter. In order to begin this exploration, I need to examine where historians have faltered.

History of Leprosy Scholarship

There is a good amount of scholarly confusion surrounding the significance of leprosy in the literature of the late Middle Ages. Part of this confusion has occurred through an oversimplification by other scholars of Saul Brody's *The Disease of the Soul: Leprosy in Medieval Literature*, a book that connected leprosy to sex in the literature of the Middle Ages. Since then, scholars have approached references to leprosy from a sexual framework, even though Brody clearly states that the association between leprosy and sin was varied and complex. Once the connection between leprosy and sex was established, scholars incorrectly applied modern medical and social connotations both to the disease and to medieval interpretations of the disease.

Interpretative problems occurred when scholars examined some of the writing of medieval doctors who claimed that leprosy could be contracted from women who recently had sex with lepers. For example, Barthelomeus Anglicus, a thirteenth-century doctor, states that leprosy "cometh of flesshely lykynge by a womman soone after that a leprous man hath laye by her" (qtd. in Brody 55). Scholars tend to approach this evidence through modern social and medical perspectives and thus explain it as describing a sexual means of transmission. Since medieval doctors declared leprosy to be contagious and believed that one could contract the disease through women, the logical inference for modern scholars is that medieval people believed leprosy was a venereal disease that punished lechery. The problem is that leprosy is not a highly contagious disease, even though medieval people believed it was, and the chances of it being transmitted venereally would be low (Brody 55–6). Furthermore, our modern concept of venereal is different from the medieval concept.

Scholars have created some interesting hypotheses in order to prove that leprosy was indeed transmitted sexually in the Middle Ages. Since we know that leprosy has a low level of transmission, some scholars assume that the medieval doctors were confused and misdiagnosed leprosy for another disease.[2] However, recent study has proven that medieval doctors were fairly accurate with their diagnosis. Hays writes:

> Although there undoubtedly occurred many misdiagnoses, medieval definitions turn out to have been remarkably good. Cemeteries known to have been set aside for 'lepers' have been exhumed, notably in Denmark, and the skeletons (or a high percentage of them) show damage of the kind caused exclusively by lepromatous leprosy; the same damage is not found in bones from other, more 'general' burial grounds. (21)

Medieval doctors did not confuse leprosy with another disease, nor did they think that leprosy was a sexually transmitted disease. The venereal hypothesis supposes instead that medieval people had a concept of disease transmission similar to ours, and that they agonized over sexually transmitted diseases. In our version of the transmission of venereal disease, a germ is passed from one person to another. Medieval doctors had no concept of the existence of these microscopic organisms. Their construction of contagious disease could therefore not be the same as ours. Instead, medieval doctors believed in a humoral system, which was influenced by sexual activity, among other things. Sometimes this sexual activity was healthy and sometimes unhealthy. The disease occurred because the humoral system of the victim was already predisposed to the disease. The action did not transfer a germ to the body but influenced what was already present in the system.

The most important idea to remember is that the disease is already present in the body of the victim, rather than coming from outside.

Brody investigates the medical, social, ecclesiastic, and literary understandings of leprosy; his examination is an important contribution to the history of the idea of disease transmission. Even though Brody's title states that he will be examining literature, only one-fifth of his book, a little over fifty pages, focuses on literature. Furthermore, within these fifty pages, Brody attempts to handle vast amounts of literature from the Anglo-Saxon to the Modern periods, and from English, German, French, and Italian sources. Further still, Brody attempts to handle a complex array of genres, from hagiography and dream visions to romances, poetry, drama, and novels. Needless to say, Brody needs to make very broad strokes to accomplish such an ambitious task. Consequently, it is difficult to apply his broad generalizations to the role of leprosy in medieval England. Whatever interpretation Brody has concerning a specific piece of literature, some counterexample from literature of a different period, time, or genre can be found to invalidate his arguments.

Brody connects leprosy and lust when he moves from "The Ecclesiastical Tradition" to his chapter on literature. Brody writes:

> While the poets received the connection of leprosy and pride solely from ecclesiastical writers, it is an oversimplification to suggest that the same sort of influence affected their use of the link between leprosy and lust. Leprosy is frequently interpreted by them as carnal sin—so frequently, in fact, that Pierre Bersuire observes that, while leprosy can signify any sin, it especially represents the sin of lust. (143)

Two clarifications of Brody's interpretation need to be addressed. First, ecclesiastical writers did not have sole ownership of the connection between leprosy and pride. Many medical writers offered moral interpretations of the disease, which they may or may not have received from ecclesiastical sources. It is not possible to identify the direct source for a moral connection to leprosy, because this connection is part of a social framework influenced and informed by a variety of social groups. Secondly, the connection between leprosy and lust is as a side-effect of the disease, not as its cause, as explicitly argued by the medical community.

The more common moral cause ascribed to leprosy are the spiritual sins, usually envy, anger, or avarice. The spiritual sins threaten the community as a whole, because sin sometimes results from not knowing one's proper social place. The medieval construction of leprosy is also connected to God. Often spiritual sins are not ones that occur as a result of interactions between men, but sins that occur as a result of interactions (or a lack of them) between man and God. Stories in multiple medieval sources describe a person who is either guilty of blasphemy or does not know his or her proper social place. God sends a disease as a sign of a sinner's threat to the faithful. The protection of the faithful by a deity could also be read politically as a desire for a lord or prince to maintain the *status quo*. Those who have social power want to maintain that power, and leprosy provided the means by which those who threatened this power structure could be isolated or removed. In this system, man's job is to recognize the sign, diagnose it as leprosy, and remove the leper from the community, thereby abating further damage to the *status quo*.

R. I. Moore was one of the first critics to read leprosy as a political and social weapon. Because leprosy is limited and specific, people can use the disease to control the morals of a society by seeking out those individuals who do not conform. In *The Formation of a Persecuting Society* (1987), Moore identified what he terms The Great Leper Hunt (c. 1090–1363). Moore develops a continuous story through an examination of the creation of hospitals and leprosariums and concludes that the statistics show "pretty unequivocally that the [Great Leper Hunt] movement began around the end of the eleventh and beginning of the twelfth centuries, surged to a peak about a hundred years later, and fell away quite quickly in the later part of the thirteenth century" (51). Moore attributes the decline in actual lepers to the ravages of the Black Death (51). But Moore does little to trace the changing beliefs about what sins lepers were accused of committing. Furthermore, while the actual number of lepers in the fourteenth century did decline, the belief system regarding lepers was kept alive by doctors, theologians, and literary authors who mythologized the disease as the ultimate punishment for transgressions against God and society.

Other historians have done more to demonstrate leprosy as a means of social control used by people in power. In *Epidemics and History: Disease, Power, and Imperialism* (1997), Sheldon Watts argues that the social climate of the eleventh century lends itself to the moralization of certain diseases, primarily as a means of social control. As Watts writes, "For religio-political authorities *circa* 1090 who hit upon the leprosy Construct as a felicitous way of ridding themselves of troublemakers, the last people they wanted meddling about were medically informed experts" (49). Watts argues that there were few secular medical experts because Salerno was just in its infancy and most doctors would have kept quiet in these unstable times in order to protect their businesses and lives (49). However, Watts fails to realize that medicine and theology were more complementary than distinct, even in Italy, let alone in England. Watts's medical hero and revolutionary, Guy de Chauliac (fl.1346–1363), also linked morality to certain illnesses, such as leprosy. Consequently, the medical community was as much a part of the "hegemonic authority" that used leprosy "as an agent of social control" as were the religious and political authorities.[3] In fact, as Watts recognizes, Guy de Chauliac was Pope Clement VI's personal physician, a job far from the fringes of the marginal, subversive society Watts wants to construct. Guy de Chauliac was part of a social system which viewed leprosy through a moral filter.

The literature of the Middle English period offers little support for the connection between the sin of lust and leprosy. Even Brody can only cite a few examples, and one is a partial misreading of Henryson's *Testament of Cresseid*. The other texts that connect leprosy to the sin of lust include French and German literary texts from the twelfth and thirteenth centuries (Brody 177–88). Brody concludes:

> In *Frauendienst*, the Tristan legend, *Jaufré*, and *The Testament of Cressid*, the leprosy is linked to physical lust; in *The Testament of Cresseid* and *Der Arme Heinrich* it punishes the sin of pride; and in the Amis and Amiloun story as in Dante, it is the consequence of falsification. In short, the association of leprosy with spiritual defilement is pervasive in the literature of the Middle Ages, and not arbitrarily so, but because common beliefs—as seen in medical, homiletic, and social attitudes—made the same connections. (189)

This list is far from the "frequent" connection Brody asserts as a transition to his chapter on literature. While an examination of French and German works that use leprosy as a punishment for lust is outside the scope of this chapter, it could be possible that different cultures believed in different causes of the same disease. Therefore, the French and German sources may proclaim leprosy as a punishment for lechery, while other people may believe that the disease punished envy or wrath. For the English, leprosy signified the spiritual sins more frequently than the carnal.

While it is true that medieval writers connected leprosy to a varied number of sins, what seems to connect all the sins together is the idea that each represented some type of falsification that threatens the community, a falsification that is connected more to language than libido. Leprosy punished people who subverted the social system for their own personal gain, such as through the sin of simony. Medieval people believed that the disease was divinely sent to identify untrustworthy or false people; therefore leprosy was seen as God's attempt to identify the people who threaten the stability of the community. In other words, leprosy is a disease that defends the community by identifying those individuals who take what is not rightfully theirs and helps the community isolate and disempower them.

Theology's View of Leprosy

In order to understand how leprosy functioned as a divinely sent disease identifying individual threats to the community, one must first examine how leprosy was understood as sent by God. The word "leprosy" has a complicated linguistic history. Leprosy seems to have reached epidemic proportions in the High Middle Ages, between the eleventh and fourteenth centuries; however, leprosy is mentioned as far back as the Greco-Roman medical corpus and in the Old Testament (Grmek 171–2). Confusion over the meaning of the word "leprosy" occurs through the translation of certain texts into other languages. The linguistic history of "leprosy" has been well documented by both historians and scholars, and I will quickly summarize how leprosy gained its moral connotations.

In Leviticus, the word "tsara'ath" which, at best, could be considered a scaly skin disease, is translated into Greek as *lepra* (Richards 9). In Greek medicine there were two different kinds of skin diseases: *lepra* and *elefantiasis*. *Lepra* could refer to a whole host of skin ailments, but *elefantiasis* meant only our modern form of leprosy or Hansen's disease. When Greek medical texts were translated into Arabic, Arabic physicians already had a name, *das fil*, which referred to many of the same ailments as *elefantiasis*. As Peter Richards argues, "This tropical disease caused by filarial worms is still known as elephantiasis today, because limbs grossly swollen and wrinkled by the disease resemble elephants' legs" (9). Since there was a disease already associated metaphorically to elephants, a new Arabic term was created to describe *elefantiasis*, *juzam*. *Juzam* was eventually translated into Latin as *lepra*, "the same word as the Greek description of a vague collection of different diseases" (Richards 9). According to Mirko Grmek, "Josephus himself translates the Biblical *Zara'at* by the term *lepra*, as does the first translation of the Pentateuch, the Septuagint, which was produced in Alexandria during the third and second centuries B.C. This is how the word 'leprosy' came into the Vulgate and acquired its medieval and modern meaning" (163). Eventually, "the Latin *lepra* and the equivalent English word leprosy acquired all the religious overtones of the Hebrew tsara'ath" (Richards 9–10). It is these religious overtones that this chapter explores. What moral connotations did the disease leprosy gain from the Bible, and how do those moral connotations influence and affect medieval society?

Stories of leprosy abound in the Old Testament. One of the most well known connections between leprosy and the clergy occurs in Leviticus 13 and 14. In Leviticus 13, the priests are given the power to diagnose skin conditions as leprous. As Brody recognizes, Leviticus's two chapters on leprosy need to be understood within the context of the book's twenty-five chapters. Brody writes, "Leviticus defines what would defile a place of worship or would keep a worshiper from entering it" (109). Consequently, chapter thirteen identifies skin conditions as clean or unclean, and chapter fourteen discusses methods by which to make a leper clean. Brody rightly recognizes that there are two categories in Leviticus:

> uncleanness of things and human uncleanness. What is common to both unclean types is that they are not holy, that is, not fit to be associated with observances in the sanctuary. It is important to recognize that uncleanness in Leviticus does not imply moral guilt: a camel is not sinful, nor is a mouse, nor a new mother, nor a house with reddish streaks, nor a leper. (110)

The same logic could be applied to Brody's supposed interpretation of the venereal nature of leprosy. In other words, sex is not unclean in itself. Instead, the uncleanness is in the location or timing of the act, be it in a church or during a woman's menstruation. The circumstances surrounding the act make it unclean and punishable by God. Leviticus does not make a direct connection between leprosy and sin, but asserts that lepers must be placed outside the community because their impurity threatens holiness and may lead others to sin or corrupt holy places.

Elsewhere in the Old Testament, leprosy is used as a means of social control, but is not of a sexual nature. The books of the Old Testament that use leprosy as a punishment focus on people who fail to know their social place and responsibilities and threaten the stability of society. These books are also markedly different from Leviticus, with its concepts of clean and unclean. Sins that threaten society are numerous, but they are not sexual. Instead, the actions of the participants are usually prideful, envious, or angry: spiritual, not carnal sins. In Numbers 12, the story of Miriam and Aaron connects leprosy to pride and envy. Miriam and Aaron speak against Moses both because he married an Ethiopian woman and because they believe themselves to be of equal stature to Moses in God's eyes. As Miriam and Aaron state, "Hath the Lord indeed spoken only by Moses? Hath he not spoken also by us?" (12:2). The Lord reprimands Miriam and Aaron by telling them that he will speak to prophets in dreams, but to the most worthy Moses, he shall speak "mouth to mouth" (12:7–8). After this reprimand, God departs turning Miriam "leprous, white as snow" (12:10). Aaron, being the priest who would confirm leprosy, quickly realizes the state of his wife and begs Moses for forgiveness: "Alas, my lord, I beseech thee, lay not the sin upon us, wherein we have done foolishly, and wherein we have sinned" (12:11). Aaron clearly sees leprosy as a reflection of a sinful state in which God's anger is reflected on the skin of Miriam. Both Miriam and Aaron envied the relationship between God and Moses. By desiring to be closer to God than they deserved, they demonstrated that they do not know their prescribed social place. The established hierarchy is that God speaks directly to Moses. He will communicate to Aaron, the priest, through dream, and never to the woman Miriam. Miriam is guilty of being envious of Moses' relationship with God.

God's reprimand comes after Miriam mischaracterizes her and Aaron's relationship to God. By arguing that the communication between God and Miriam is the same as that between Moses and God, Miriam attempts to portray herself as Moses' equal. God corrects this blasphemy with the punishment of leprosy. After Moses asks for Miriam to be healed, the Lord emphasizes the importance of knowing one's social place by saying, "If her father had but spit in her face, should she not be ashamed seven days? let her be shut out from the camp seven days, and after that let her be received in again" (12:15). The Lord punishes Miriam with leprosy and exile because she is twice guilty of not knowing her social position. She is first guilty of attempting to make herself Moses' equal; and second, she is a woman trying to usurp the intermediary role of a priest between God and man, a role reserved for men. In other words, Miriam attempts to usurp two social positions—first a man and then a priest or a prophet.

II Chronicles 26 also demonstrates God's punishment of individuals who do not know their social place. However, what makes II Chronicles 26 interesting is that the sins surrounding leprosy also include anger. Uzziah, a powerful king and ruler, desires to celebrate his fortune at war by burning incense in the temple. The priests of the temple admonish Uzziah, telling him, "It appertaineth not unto thee Uzziah, to burn incense unto the Lord, but to the priests the sons of Aaron, that are consecrated to burn incense: go out of the sanctuary; for thou hast trespassed; neither shall it be for thine honour from the Lord God" (26:18).

Uzziah does not heed the priest's orders; instead, he "was wroth, and had a censer in his hand to burn incense: and while he was wroth with the priests, the leprosy even rose up in his forehead before the priests in the Lord, from beside the incense altar" (26:19). Like Miriam, Uzziah is guilty of attempting to better his social position by performing actions that only the priests are allowed to perform. His anger is prominently displayed as the cause of his leprosy, but equal emphasis should be placed on his attempt to falsely identify himself as a priest. Unlike Miriam, Uzziah does not repent his sins and he receives no cure; instead, he spends the rest of his life exiled as a leper, "cut off from the house of the Lord" (26:21). The story of Uzziah points to the necessity of contrition for a sinner to be cured. Aaron recognizes his and Miriam's sins and asks for God's forgiveness. Uzziah, on the other hand, fails to admit his sins; therefore, he remains a threat to the stability of the social order and must be expelled from the community. What is being threatened is the hierarchy between God and man. Only certain people are allowed to communicate with God. Both Miriam and Uzziah are envious of the priest's position in relation to God.

Leprosy also functions in the Old Testament as a means of punishment for avarice, particularly simony. In II Kings 5, Naaman, captain to the King of Syria, is described as a great man, "but he was a leper" (5:1). Naaman suffers from anger and pride, and he lacks faith in God. An Israeli captive becomes the maid for Naaman's wife and tells her that there is a great prophet in the land of Samaria that could cure Naaman's leprosy (5:2–3). Desiring a cure, Naaman asks the King of Syria to seek out this prophet and provides the King with numerous gifts as an incentive to purchase Naaman's salvation. The King tears at his clothes because he is not a God who "can kill and make . . . alive" (5:7). This line clearly demonstrates the divine associations of this disease. Leprosy makes a living person dead in the eyes of the Church and God. Thus to be able to cure leprosy would, in a sense, be the ability to bring one back from the dead. Elisha comes to the King's rescue by saying that he can cure Naaman. When Naaman arrives at Elisha's door, Elisha sends a messenger to tell Naaman to "wash in Jordan seven times" (5:10). Namaan becomes angry because he desires a different type of consultation: "He will surely come out to me, and stand, and call on the name of the Lord his God, and strike his hand over the place, and recover the leper" (5:11). Naaman's anger and his pride, demonstrated by his desire to be treated on equal social terms rather than being dealt with by a messenger, illustrate the flaws in his character which the leprosy is punishing.

It is Naaman's servant who corrects the captain by saying, "My father, if the prophet had bid thee do some great thing, wouldest thou have done it? how much rather then, when he saith to thee, Wash, and be clean?" (5:13). Naaman takes his servant's advice and dips himself in Jordan and becomes clean. Naaman returns to Elisha and says, "Behold, now I know that there is no God in all the earth, but in Israel: now therefore, I pray thee, take a blessing of thy servant" (5:15). Naaman's words demonstrate that he has both lost his anger and accepts his inferior social position to that of the priest and God. Consequently, his leprosy is healed.

II Kings 5 continues with Elisha refusing the blessing of Naaman, and Naaman stating that he will only give blessings and offerings to the Lord as a result of his cure (5:15–19). These offerings cause another character, Gehazi, to be punished with leprosy, because he commits the sin of avarice. Elisha's servant, Gehazi, rides after the departing Naaman and says, "My master hath sent me, saying, Behold, even now there be come to me from mount Ephraim two young men of the sons of the prophets: give them, I pray thee, a talent of silver, and two changes of garments" (5:22). Naaman does this and Gehazi hides the money and clothes in Elisha's house. Elisha immediately questions Gehazi saying, "Is it a time to receive money, and to receive garments . . . the leprosy therefore of Naaman shall cleave unto thee, and unto thy seed for ever" (5:26–7). Gehazi is guilty of avarice, particularly simony, because he tried to make a personal gain from God's cure. He is punished with leprosy, the very disease he attempted to profit from.

The Old Testament stories that include leprosy as a punishment for sin revolve around four of the spiritual sins: pride, envy, anger, and avarice. These are sins that seem to threaten the relationship between God and man because the sinner does not know his or her rightful social place in God's hierarchy. Miriam is stricken with leprosy because she is envious of Moses and God's relationship, and she commits blasphemy as she tries to subvert both divine order between God and Moses and domestic order between man and woman. Likewise, Uzziah attempts to overtake the social role of the priests in relation to burning incense. Finally, Naaman learns his social position as inferior to Elisha and thereby is cleansed of his pride and anger. Gehazi fails to realize his social position both as a servant of Elisha and the Lord and commits avarice as he attempts to sell God's gifts. Consequently, Elisha punishes Gehazi for his sin of avarice, specifically simony, through the disfigurement of leprosy. In the works of the Old Testament, leprosy is a disease sent down by God that punishes transgressors who threaten social order and stability. Once the disease is identified, these people are removed from the community into outposts, thereby protecting the community from their further infections, both of a physical and social nature.

Leprosy's relation to religious hierarchy is also evident in theological writers of the thirteenth and fourteenth centuries. In *Handlyng Synne* (1303), Robert Mannyng of Brunne creates "a long poem on the fundamentals of Christian religion, illustrated with many stories and *exempla*" (Bloomfield 171). A large part of the work investigates the Seven Deadly Sins; however, he does not mention leprosy in relation to the sins. Instead he mentions leprosy in relation to penance, particularly shrift. Mannyng's mention of leprosy is metaphoric, but what is interesting is that once he mentions it, he is automatically led to ideas related to proper social relations and meekness. In the fourth point of shrift, Mannyng states that "mekenes ys so noble a ȝyfte" (11463). Meekness seems to be the controlling idea as Mannyng describes the way a leper came to Jesus and was healed by him because of the leper's "myldenes" (11471). Mannyng explains,

> He þat ys yn dedly synne,
> Gostly, he ys a mesel wyþ ynne.
> He þat wyl hys hele seke,
> To hys prest he mote be meke. (11473–76)

In this passage, leprosy (the mesel) is used metaphorically to describe the state of one's soul suffering from deadly sin. To cleanse the leprous soul, one needs to know one's social position and humble one's self in front of those who are socially better, the priests. Mannyng's use of leprosy is similar to the story of Naaman who desires to have the priest perform the cleansing according to Naaman's own wishes. Mannyng states that the only way to cleanse sin is to be truthful to the priest, just as the only way to cleanse leprosy is to listen the priest's directions.[4]

In the *Parson's Tale*, Chaucer connects leprosy to the sins of chiding and reproach under the larger sin of anger. Under the topic of anger, the Parson states, "Lat us thanne speken of chidynge and reproache, which been ful grete woundes in mannes herte, for they unsowen the semes of freendshipe in mannes herte" (X.621). The sin of reproach causes hostility between men of the community: "For certes, unnethes may a man pleynly been accorded with hym that hath openly revyled and repreved and disclaundred. This is a ful grisly synne, as Christ seith in the gospel" (X.622). If someone chides or reproaches another person, he or she apparently does not know his or her proper social place. It is only God's place to chide or reproach men.

Often people chide or reproach others because the other has a sign or symptom that differentiates him or her from the majority. The Parson states, "And taak kep now, that he that repreveth his neighebor, outher he repreveth hym by som harm of peyne that he hath on his body, as 'mesel,' 'croked harlot,' or some synne that he dooth" (X.623). In other words, one should avoid using clear signs, such as leprosy, to continue to punish those stricken with the disease. The Parson is not saying that it is socially acceptable to admonish these individuals no matter how imbued in sin they are. Instead, the Parson asks Christians to "turneth the repreve to Jhesu Crist, for peyne is sent by the rightways sonde of God, and by his suffrance, be it meselrie, mayheym, or maladie" (X.624). The Parson advocates a new form of charity whereby the reproach is left to God rather than left among the people. The leper's disease is the "suffrance" the sinner pays for the sin. It is not necessary for man to punish the leper also. What cannot be ignored in this passage is that leprosy is divinely sent both as a punishment and as a means of identifying those being punished by God.

The *Parson's Tale* demonstrates a positive social role for lepers that can also be traced back to the Bible. In the New Testament, Jesus cures a leper in three of the four gospels: Matthew 8:2–4, Mark 1:40–45, and Luke 5:12–16. Only Mark adds that the cured leper does not listen to Christ's advice to keep the miracle a secret (1:44–5). Interestingly, Jesus and the leper seem to switch social places, for as Mark declares, "Jesus could no longer enter a town openly but stayed outside in lonely places" (1:45).[5] Nevertheless, Jesus' work with lepers changes the social position and power of the lepers. While they still remain the outcasts of society, lepers also become the medium for good deeds and salvation for both the lay and the clerical populations. Watts sums up this paradox: "Though a leper could be seen as a representative of Christ offering opportunities for Christian charity, the leper was also seen as a sin-curst being who, following the precepts of Leviticus must be cast out of the community of the faithful" (52). In *Piers Plowman*, William Langland places lepers within a host of other social groups, such as the old, women and children, prisoners, and pilgrims. Leprosy is the only disease listed within this group, whose members have the potential to better the human spirit. Truth states, "For loue of here lowe hertes oure lord hath hem ygraunted / Here penaunce and here purgatorye vppon this puyre erthe" (V.184–5). The leper becomes someone to envy because his or her penance and purgatory is performed on earth.

The status of lepers also improved, at least theoretically, when biblical confusion over the identity of Lazarus resulted in interpretations which argued that lepers are tormented on the earthly plane but will receive immediate heavenly salvation. Richards explains the exegetical confusion: "By some strange and tortuous thinking, Lazarus the beggar became identified with Lazarus of Bethany, whom Jesus raised from the dead, conveniently perhaps, for it may have seemed to promise certain resurrection to the lepers" (8). Nevertheless, even with the improvement of the leper's social and afterlife positioning, leprosy still represented the spiritual sins, primarily sins which relate to God's relationship and communication with man.

Leprosy represents a conservative desire to read the disease as a form of social control in order to maintain the *status quo*. Consequently, one of the roles of the caretakers of society is to remain vigilant to the signs of leprosy because God is identifying certain people as a threat to the social order and community. These people accordingly should be expelled from the community to protect the social order until God heals their leprosy.

THE MEDICAL COMMUNITY'S INTERPRETATION OF LEPROSY

Beliefs expressed about leprosy through biblical sources are similar to those found in medical manuscripts of the late Middle Ages. The medieval medical community was part of a social system that believed in a relationship between morality and disease. This examination will demonstrate that for the medieval medical doctor uncontrollable sexuality was a side effect of leprosy, not a cause, and that medicine and theology focused on the leper as a person who is both unclean and threatens the society.

Medieval physicians and surgeons often describe the effects of disease through humoral imbalances. While leprosy might seem to be untreatable in the Middle Ages, many surgical manuals have passages on how to diagnosis and treat leprosy. This points to a medical hierarchy in which doctors, who sat at the top, may not have wanted to treat lepers, and therefore left the treatment to those of lesser prestige. While a modern reader might not expect leprosy to be a topic of a surgery textbook, one must keep in mind that surgery was considered to be a general craft, not an institutionalized specialization. Numerous attempts were made to institutionalize surgery through guilds, but all failed under the weight and power of the Barber's Guild. Eventually, surgeons allied themselves with the Barber's Guild in 1540 (Beck 125). For university-trained authors like Lanfrank, the idea that surgery was a craft that did not require significant learning was appalling. Consequently, Lanfrank argues that the surgeon should be "so lerne ... [in] fisik, pat he mowe wiþ good rulis his surgerie defende & þat techip fisik! Nepeles it is nessessarie a surgian to knowe allen þe parties and ech sengle partie of a medicyn" (9). For Lanfrank, surgeons must know both medicine and surgery to perform adequately. Therefore, it is of little surprise that Lanfrank would include a discussion of leprosy in his surgical textbooks.

In the earliest vernacular edition of Lanfrank of Milan's[6] *Chirguria Magna*, the author describes how leprosy develops.[7] Lanfrank begins his chapter on leprosy by stating that the disease "comep of malancolie corrupt" (196). One of the four humors, melancholy, is associated with the earth and is considered to be both dry and cold. Nearly all medieval doctors and surgeons believed that leprosy is caused by corrupted melancholy. Even though leprosy has a physiological cause, the disease itself does not preclude moral associations or divine visitations. For example, in *The Anatomy of Melancholy* (1621),[8] Robert Burton writes, "God himself is a cause [of melancholy], for the punishment of sin and satisfaction of his justice, many examples & testimonies of holy Scriptures make evident unto us" (156). While Burton is writing in the seventeenth century, it is clear that, through the Renaissance and Enlightenment, there was still a sense that even if the physical reasons for an ailment are known, the disease might nevertheless be divinely sent. To this day, we still distinguish between a distant and a proximate cause: people ask the question, "What did I do to deserve this?" when faced with a disease or accident. Medieval people were no less reflective on the nature of illness.

Modern scientific sensibilities recognize a paradox between natural and divine causes of disease. However, a different social framework structured the medieval mind. According to Amundsen, medieval Europe "striv[ed] to subordinate medicine in all its aspects of religion":

> This is not to suggest that medieval European ecclesiastics wished to impose religious nosology and therapeutic models. Indeed, their understanding of disease was essentially naturalistic, and their therapies were typically naturalistic as well. But their belief in the sovereignty of God as the Final Cause, in his freedom to intervene in natural processes, and in the subtle trickery of evil powers that draw people away from God by healing them directly or luring them to rely on naturalistic models without reference to, or dependence on, Him, motivated ecclesiastical authorities throughout the Middle Ages to subordinate medicine to the prevailing Christian construct of reality and to Christian ethics. (2–3)

It is possible, therefore, to have a natural explanation for disease, to even know the physical causes of the disease, *and* to also believe in divine causality. The medical and theological construction of certain diseases, for example leprosy, demonstrates both natural and divine reasons for the disease. The natural explanations focus on a corrupted melancholy, while the divine argues that a person is melancholic because he or she is morally corrupt.

Many of the moral associations listed in medical and surgical manuals of the Middle Ages are designed to help doctors diagnose a disease. While many of the observations are relatively free of moral judgment (for example, salty or greasy blood was believed to be common to lepers), more interesting for my purposes are descriptions that are value-laden and focus on a moral connection between leprosy and sin. As Brody rightly points out, in the eleventh century, Theodoric states that lepers "grow angry very easily, and more easily than was customary. Evil, crafty habits appear; patients suspect everyone of wanting to hurt them" (51). In the late thirteenth century, Roland's *Cyrurgia* states that lepers have "mores mali," bad morals (Singer, "Thirteenth Century," 238). Similarly, Guy du Chauliac points out that lepers "ben rowhe and ful of akþe and full wood, and þay wil presye hemself ouer mykel among þe people" (380). Consequently, Chauliac states that the physician should "enquere ham of þe things or tokens þat þai knowe, and þerwiþ of here queyntise and of her maners and of here dremes and here desires" (381).[9] Obviously the medical community believed in a moral association of this disease.

Luke Demaitre disagrees with the view that medieval doctors subscribed to a moral connotation of disease. This view "lures [historians] into inferring that medieval physicians sanctioned the moral overtones which indisputably dominated the treatment of leprosy in the literary, devotional, and popular sources" (336). In other words, Demaitre wants to believe that medieval doctors are free from the lenses by which their society constructs disease. While everyone else interprets leprosy from a moral framework, doctors, claims Demaitre, are free of that purportedly narrow vision. It is hard to see how medieval doctors did not interpret leprosy as a moral disease when the three sins doctors identified with leprosy—anger, envy, and avarice—are the same three sins connected to leprosy in the Old Testament.

Even the medical community advanced the notion that lepers are falsifiers and deceivers who have the potential to threaten the community. Chauliac declares, "þat is þe most iniurie (i. wrong) to sequestre or wiþdrawe þo men þat schulde not be sequestered or wiþdrawen and leue leprouse men with þe peple" (381). Sheldon Watts points out that in this comment Chauliac demonstrates a new type of health care, a more humane and less political medical system because Chauliac is concerned about misdiagnosis that Watts believes was often committed by civic authorities for their own political ends (58). But Watts only quotes the first part concerning sequestering healthy men, but leaves out the ending part: "or wiþdrawen and leue leprouse men with þe peple." Evidently the second part of Chauliac's quote implies some type of threat to the community if lepers are not identified and removed. Identifying what type of threat lepers pose to the community is problematic. While the spiritual sins are most evident in Chauliac's work, he also states that lepers should try to abstain from sexual acts. The abstinence from sex points not to leprosy as a venereal disease, but as a side-effect to disease itself.

When discussing the venereal nature of diseases in the Middle Ages, we need to be careful to deal with the disease on their terms, not ours. The word "venereal," meaning a communicable disease contracted through sexual intercourse, was not used until 1658, and it was then associated with syphilis. Demaitre states, "While the notions of susceptibility and continued exposure may soften the contrast between our own understanding and the medieval descriptions of leprosy as congenital and contagious, the venereal aspects remain irreconcilable with modern findings that the disease is not transmitted sexually" (334). Modern doctors know that leprosy does not have a venereal means of transmission, even though medieval doctors seem to have believed that it did. This irreconcilable finding has led many medical historians to assume that medieval doctors were using the term "leprosy" as an umbrella term for syphilis, even though there is significant documentation that syphilis was not present in its venereal form in the Middle Ages.[10]

What may be more likely is that medieval doctors did not mean that leprosy was a venereal disease in our modern terminology. During the fourteenth and fifteenth centuries, "venereal" was associated with overt sexual desire or sexual intercourse. In this time period, doctors believed in a humoral system which could be influenced by certain physical actions. The disease is already present in the body of the person and is brought out through improper actions. The fourteenth-century definition implies a problem with the person's moral nature; it is an internal problem.

Within the word "venereal" lie two different linguistic associations: "venial," meaning "sin," and "venery," meaning "sex." Claude Quétel describes the moral connotations of "venereal":

> These two [syphilis and gonorrhea], which are popularly christened 'the pox' and 'the clap,' as if to tame them, have been practically the only diseases of the human race to be named according to the means by which they are transmitted: venereal. The word carries connotation of both sex and sin. One is punished by the very means in which one has transgressed. (3)

Most modern scholars have confused the reason that medical doctors declare that lepers burn for sex and that the disease can be transmitted through women who have lain with a leper. These two ideas are totally separate, and neither is venereal in our modern terminology. Furthermore, the role of women in the transmission of leprosy remains highly complex and problematic. At some level, according to medieval medical information, women tend to have a limited immunity to the disease because of their colder, moister bodies; nevertheless, they can still contract the disease. Examining the humoral framework medieval doctors applied to diseases such as leprosy can solve the problems of interpreting this disease.

For the Middle Ages, disease transmission is a process by which a certain act influences a humoral imbalance in the person affected. In modern disease pathology, germs are passed from one person to another through cellular membranes. Consequently, leprosy cannot be associated with our form of venereal transmission because germs are not passing from one person to another. Instead, the act, in this case sexual, influences the humoral system and brings about the disease. The body, for medieval people, is a closed system that can be affected by the outside forces. Disease can also be seen as divinely sent, since God could influence the humors especially if He were punishing an unclean or inappropriate sexual act. Although medieval doctors paid particular attention to women who had recent intercourse with a leper, this does not point to a venereal nature of leprosy. The woman would not have leprosy, but instead would have fluid from a leper that could influence other fluids, and, in turn, affect the humoral system of the next man she had intercourse with. In modern terms, a woman is infected and infects another man by passing a germ to him. In medieval terms, the woman influences the humoral balance in the second man because she has the leper's fluid inside her. This humoral influence brings about leprosy in the second lover. The major difference is that in our system the disease comes from outside the body and both the female and the male are infected, whereas in the medieval system the disease is in the body awaiting a propitious balance of humors before emerging.

Lanfrank writes that lepers "wilineþ myche to comne wiþ wommen" (197). Similarly, Roland says, "Ardent plurimi eorum in coytu," (most burn for sex) (Singer, "Thirteenth Century," 239). The connection between lepers and a desire for sex is not a condemnation of the sexual act by the medical establishment, nor is it demonstrative of a connection between the moral nature of the disease and the person infected. Rather the connection between leprosy and increased sexual desire comes directly from humoral theory. In *Sexuality and Medicine in the Middle Ages*, Danielle Jacquart and Claude Thomasset argue:

> The treatise of Ishâ ibn-'Imrân, translated in the eleventh century by Constantine the African under the title *De Melancholia*, spread two ideas that were frequently developed: on the one hand, too rigorously an ascetic life risks causing the illness of melancholy; on the other hand, this illness can find relief thanks to coitus. Likewise the Canon of Avicenna cites among the benefits of the sexual act; the 'expulsion' of a dominant train of thought or of an obsession, the acquisition of boldness, the control of excessive anger and, of course, the dissolution of the spermatic vapours that accumulate in the brain of melancholics. (83)

Through logical indirection, if sufferers of melancholy could find relief from their ailment through coitus, and if doctors believed that leprosy developed out of a corrupted form of melancholy, then it would make sense that lepers desired sexual contact as a result and possible relief from their disease. Lanfrank does not condemn the desire for coitus; rather it is simply part of his list that he gives fellow doctors so that they can diagnose the presence of the disease.

Bernard de Gordon (c. 1285–1308) and his student, Guy de Chauliac, come the closest to prohibiting sexual intercourse for lepers. According to Demaitre: "Bernard taught that, contrary to 'the common belief (*vulgaris opinio*) that coitus is not only beneficial but even therapeutic for leprosy, it is not advisable because all lepers are radically cold and dry as a result of the disease's nature'—and, of course, sex had a drastic cooling and drying effect" (339). Along similar lines, Chauliac writes, "And ouer þoo, þai schal eschewe fro leccherye and fro all þing pat may chaufe here nature, as Avicen saith" (385). Chauliac prohibits sex not because leprosy is venereal and can be transmitted from person to person, but because lechery could adversely change the humoral system. Lechery is desiring others physically, and the desire would shake up the leper's humors. Once again, Chauliac demonstrates how morality affects the body. Further, Chauliac is not prescribing abstinence; rather he is describing a sinful behavior, a behavior that makes one unclean. In other words, the leper is permitted to have sex with his or her spouse because that is morally proper.

In *Fasciculus Morum: A Fourteenth-Century Preacher's Handbook*, the author describes the nature of lechery:

> Ipsa autem tamquam publica meretrix cum nullo veretur commisceri; unde merito execrabilis iudicatur. Secundo de eius contrario, scilicet de continencia et puritate cum suis membris. (648)
>
> Like a public whore, this vice is not ashamed to lie with anybody; whence it is rightly deemed to be accursed. Following it, we will deal with its opposite virtue, namely continence and purity, its members. (Trans. Siegfried Wenzel 649)

Sexual activity or intercourse is not lechery as long as the person is monogamous. Lechery, as defined by the *Fasciculus*, is desiring to have extramarital intercourse with others. The leper is not permitted to have sex with numerous partners or to desire other people because that would constitute lechery. Because no medical doctor declares intercourse off limits, the leper may have sex with his rightful partner. Even the Third Lateran Council (1179) had priests declare to lepers: "I forbid [you] to live with any woman other than your own" (qtd. in Hays 23). Obviously the leper was allowed to have sexual relations with his own wife, but not have lecherous desire for other people. The connection between leprosy and lechery is a prohibition that reflects more on medieval social mores than on a belief in a venereal means of disease transmission.

Leprosy is transmitted because the lecherous desire already exists in an individual's body, and if the right set of circumstances happens, namely sex with a woman who has recently lain with a leper, then this act may bring about the humoral situation by which leprosy manifests itself. According to many medical works, leprosy is transmitted through a woman if she has had sex with a leprous man prior to the sexual contact with the second man. For example, Roland argues that those "who are infected from sex with a woman who had coitus with a leper" suffer from an irregular heartbeat (Singer "Thirteenth Century" 239).[11] Furthermore, Bernard de Gordon in *Lillum Medicine* (1303) writes, "Everyone ought to guard against lying with a leperous woman, and I will tell what happened: a certain countess came leprous to Montpellier, and in the end she was under my treatment. A bachelor of medicine who attended to her lay with her and impregnated her, and he was made completely leperous" (qtd. in Demaitre 330). It would appear that Bernard implies that there is some form of venereal transmission occurring in this anecdote, and certain medical historians have put a lot of weight on these lines as evidence of medieval doctors diagnosing syphilis for leprosy.

However, Demaitre has shown that Bernard's ideas were not transferred to his student, Guy du Chauliac, or shared by Bernard's peers. Demaitre writes:

> It is ironic that Guy's omission [of sex as the cause of leprosy] sorely irked and disappointed Holcomb, who complained that everything Bernard had 'told us of the venereal features was ignored and lost through the influence of one who occupied a dangerous position of authority; being physician to three Popes ... Guy de Chauliac ignored the importance of *primitive* or external causes such are the result of the dangers of contact infection through venery.' (335)

The medical faculty that surrounded Bernard also failed to mention sex as a cause of leprosy. Demaitre writes, "It is particularly significant that no allusion to sex as a cause was made by Arnald de Villanova, Bernard de Gordon's senior colleague at Montpellier, in his treatise *On the Examination of Lepers*, or by Jordanus de Turre, a successor of Bernard in the 1320s, in his *Notes on Leprosy*" (335). Bernard's anecdote may simply be a medical enigma that he felt the need to document, or it may point to a specific cultural belief about the power of diseased women.

The connection between women and leprosy created some very heated debates in medical schools. Jacquart and Thomasset describe the most common question asked of medical teachers, such as William of Conches, concerning this ailment: "Why, if a leper knows a woman, is the woman left unharmed, whereas the first man to know her thereafter will become a leper?" (189). William responds:

> The hottest woman is colder than the coldest man: such a complexion is hard and extremely resistant to male corruption; nonetheless the putrid matter, coming from coitus with lepers remains in the womb. And when a man penetrates her the penis, made of sinews, enters the vagina (vulva) and, by virtue of its attractive force, attracts this matter to itself (and to the organs to which it is attached) and transmits it to them. (qtd. in Jacquart and Thomasset 189)

Jacquart and Thomasset defend this interpretation by both finding a venereal disease, *lymphogranuloma venereum*, that could actually be transmitted from woman to man and arguing that medieval women would not have had the freedom that men had; therefore they had less possibility of contraction.

In opposition to Jacquart and Thomasset, I suggest that the imagined immunity of women to leprosy fits a cultural model thoroughly examined by feminists. In *Poison Damsels and Other Essays in Folklore and Anthropology*, N. M. Penzer traces the woman-as-polluter theme in literature. One of the more common cultural themes, for example, is the woman who has a *vagina dentata*, a vagina with teeth, which castrates men (41–44). Through an expansion of Penzer's work, Barbara Fass Leavy argues "[t]hat gynecological disorders and venereal diseases may contribute to such tales adds a fascinatingly realistic layer of meaning to what is a virtually endlessly provocative symbolism" (170). Penzer's study examines the ways in which different cultures create myths about immune but contagious women who spread syphilis to unsuspecting men (44–71). Penzer concludes, "I would say that the *motif* of the poison-damsel originated in India at a very early period before the Christian era. The poison-damsel herself has no existence in actual fact, but is merely the creation of the story-teller, who derived the idea from what he saw around him" (71). The arguments presented by medieval doctors about the contagious nature of leprosy fit this common cultural myth, justified primarily by the authority of medicine. After a woman laid with a leper, she could infect another man for a certain period of time because the second man's humoral system was predisposed to leprosy. The fluid within the woman did not infect the man in the modern sense of disease transmission, but rather influenced the humoral system of the man who is hotter and drier. Because the woman is moister and colder, her humoral system is left unharmed. Thus, the woman can pollute others in the society without ever suffering from the disease.

At least from a medical standpoint, sex is not wrong in the Middle Ages, because it is necessary for health. Further, sex does not bring about leprosy; rather, lechery is wrong and can influence the emergence of the disease if one desires too much. According to medieval doctors, disease was an imbalance of the humors; therefore, leprosy, in a sense, was already present in the body but simply needed the right influence to bring the disease about. The interpretation of the disease by the medical and theological community demonstrates a form of social control, primarily the control of the *status quo*. Lepers were believed to be guilty of one of the spiritual sins, pride, envy wrath, or avarice. When leprosy was connected to sexuality, it either related to the side effects a leper experienced, such as uncontrolled sexual desire, or the influence of the humoral system in an already sinful body. Leprosy's connection to sex is a means of social control, a control endorsed by the medical community to keep people from desiring other people who are not rightfully theirs.

Scholars and historians need to be careful how they interpret beliefs about contagion in the Middle Ages, especially in relation to venereal diseases. Leprosy's means of transmission in the Middle Ages seems to partake in the more common cultural motif of the poison damsel than in the notion that medical doctors had some rudimentary idea of pathogens. More importantly, the moral connections medieval people made with respect to leprosy reflect their own social and communal fears. Medieval doctors, laypersons, and clergy believed, at some level, that leprosy was a punishment sent by God for an individual's sins.

Responding to the Plague

The connection between sin and disease became even more evident when the bubonic plague struck. The moral system that doctors and theologians used to interpret leprosy was also used to interpret the plague. However, since plague was an acute disease that struck numerous people and since there was no biblical source for plague, medieval people interpreted the disease as a punishment for an all-encompassing sin, Pride. This interpretation gave all the power and control of the disease to God, for only He would know when enough people had forsaken Pride so that the plague could end. Like leprosy, this epidemic disease was totally in the hands of God, and all man could do was to try to repent. Eventually, man realized that the end of the world was not coming, and he could develop protective measures against plague. These protective measures do not mean that people interpreted the moral meaning of the disease differently. What it does show is an attempt to exert some kind of control on the judgments of God, even if limited.

The Rand Corporation ranks the Black Death as the third worst catastrophe to affect the world (Gottfried, *Black Death*, xiv).[12] From 1347 to 1351, the Black Death killed twenty-five to fifty percent of Europe's population (Gottfried, *Black Death*, xiii). Subsequent outbreaks occurred between 1349 and 1450 and further reduced the population from 1347 to between sixty and seventy-five percent (Gottfried, *Black Death*, 133).[13] As our society struggles with its own versions of plague, namely HIV and AIDS, it is relatively easy to empathize with our medieval counterparts' feeling of helplessness. To refer again to Sontag's metaphor, the bubonic plague that struck Europe provided both a new passport to and a new region of the kingdom of the ill. The birth of a new disease or kingdom provides two important theoretical problems. First, one needs to interpret the disease morally. If one believes that God sent down the disease to correct the wicked, what sin is it that God wants to correct? Unlike leprosy, which appeared in the Bible, bubonic plague had no authoritative history to guide the people to understand the meaning of this disease. Secondly, the main difference between plague and other diseases is that plague strikes large groups of people rather than individuals. Consequently, the passport for individuals entering the plague kingdom would not necessarily be stamped with the correct moral qualifications associated with this disease. Medieval authorities had to explain how these relatively spiritually pure people stood beside the guilty as they were led into the kingdom of plague.

AIDS is a modern-day example of the problems that occur in an interpretative system in which there are two kingdoms and the members of one kingdom are associated with a specific sin believed to cause their disease. Even before the medical community identified the new Human Immunodeficiency Virus (HIV), some groups interpreted HIV and AIDS as a punishment sent by God to correct sexual promiscuity, homosexuality, and drug use. In this interpretative structure, People With AIDS (PWAs) brought the disease on themselves through immoral actions. Once one constructs this type of interpretative framework, what does one do with the innocent sufferers of the disease? For example, how does one explain the children who are born with HIV and the hemophiliacs who need blood, but receive infected stock? Moreover, in this framework, how does one know which sin God is attempting to correct? Is it drug use or promiscuity, homosexuality or lechery? When we create dichotomies such as these, the definitions of the groups being punished become extremely problematic. For example, in many cases, heterosexual couples practice the same sexual acts as homosexual couples, namely anal and oral sex. According to this framework then, homosexuality would be defined, at some level, not as what homosexuals do, but as what they cannot perform, namely vaginal intercourse. So if the disease punishes a sexual act, why does it not punish heterosexuals as well as homosexuals? Or does it punish promiscuity, regardless of the gender of the sexual participants? Medieval people struggled with similar interpretative questions when faced with bubonic plague: what sin does this disease identify and why are the innocent punished alongside the guilty? It is the latter question, I believe, that forces people to abandon the dichotomy of healthy and ill and accept a disease as a new part of life.

By examining the construction of and tracking the references to plague in medieval writings, one can observe a method of coping by which the disease is initially read as a punishment for sin and scapegoats are sought. The reason for the disease is essentially sought outside the community. Eventually, the disease becomes a part of the fabric of human life and the references to the disease become metaphoric. As Michael Dols cautions, "The most important thing to bear in mind [when discussing plague] is not the precise mechanisms contrived by men to explain contagion (which were wrong) but the fact that in the Middle Ages—whether in Christian or in Muslim society—one simply could not separate the physiological from the mental and moral process" (286). More importantly, one must remember that theories of plague are only incorrect upon retrospect. For medieval authors, these theories were founded on the most current information of the time.

History of Bubonic Plague Scholarship

The bubonic plague is one of the more carefully studied areas in the history of medicine. Robert Gottfried's *The Black Death: Natural and Human Disaster in Medieval Europe* (1983) includes an excellent bibliographic essay (187–194). Instead of duplicating Gottfried's work, I will focus on the books that are important to the understanding of the bubonic plague as a social event and examine the works that came after Gottfried's publication. Many historians point to an environmental cause of the outbreak of bubonic plague, and both Hans Zinsser and Robert Gottfried offer examples of the type of work being done in this field. In *Rats, Lice, and History* (1934), Zinsser writes "to impress the fact that we are dealing with a phase of man's history on earth which has received too little attention from poets, artists, and historians. Swords and lances, arrows, machine guns, and even high explosives have had far less power over the fates of nations than the typhus louse, the plague flea, and the yellow-fever mosquito" (9). Zinsser discusses the ways these three diseases are altered by environmental conditions. Concerning the bubonic plague, Zinsser rightly recognizes that while at least one-quarter of the European population, nearly 25 million, died in the first plague outbreak, the numbers of fatalities declined considerably over subsequent visitations. Zinsser writes, "In 1348, two thirds of the population were afflicted, and almost all died; in 1362, half the population contracted the disease and very few survived; in 1371, only one tenth were sick, and many survived; while in 1382, only one twentieth of the population became sick, and almost all survived" (89). Zinsser attributes the change in mortality not to increased immune resistance, nor to better medical care, but rather to changes in environment. The most important reason why we no longer see major outbreaks of bubonic plague in civilized countries, according to Zinsser, is because rats are domesticated and "do not migrate through cities and villages as they formerly did" (93). Nevertheless, Zinsser's study does not explain how over a period of less than 40 years, the mortality of humans to bubonic plague changed from two-thirds to less than ten percent. The rat could not be domesticated this quickly. Furthermore, because of drastic improvement in survival rates, one can definitely see how medieval people would have maintained faith in their medical community.

In *The Black Death: Natural and Human Disaster in Medieval Europe* (1983), Robert Gottfried offers one answer as to how the mortality improved over such a short time period. As Gottfried writes, "The Black Death and the second plague pandemic can be understood only in their epidemiological context, as part of a 300-year period of ecological crisis" (xvi). Gottfried studies human conditions, such as trade routes and civic regulations, in combination with changes in rodent communities through climate studies. What Gottfried finds is that the fleas took to human food sources only after they diminished their primary food source, the black rat. "In effect," Gottfried writes, "humans are victims of changes in insect and rodent ecology" (*Black Death*, 7). As rural areas were abandoned and people headed to towns, the abandoned areas went back to forest and pasturelands, enabling an environmental balance to occur (Gottfried, *Black Death*, 135). The second plague pandemics kept the human population low, thereby preventing another major outbreak (Gottfried, *Black Death*, 156).

Besides environmental studies of the Black Death, historians have examined how the Black Death's mortality changed social institutions. Colin Platt's *King Death: The Black Death and Its Aftermath in Late-Medieval England* (1997) explores many of the social changes brought about by the bubonic plague, focusing mainly on the economic. Platt writes, "What the Black Death began was a severe labour shortage which persisted little changed for a century and more, and which was not entirely over even then" (viii). Platt examines how the bubonic plague changed inheritance practices, the role of gentry, family structure, and marriages. Platt finds that the plague gave people economic and social freedoms that were unknown to the lower classes in the pre-plague years (192).

The latest works to examine the importance of bubonic plague to social history are David Herlihy's *The Black Death* (1997) and Jo Hays's *The Burdens of Disease* (1998). Herlihy's book consists of three essays that were given at the University of Maine and were found after Herlihy's death. Introduced by Samuel Cohen, the three studies examine the bubonic plague as the turning point from a medieval to modern sensibility (4). One of the three essays reexamines Graham Twigg's theory, published in *The Black Death: A Biological Reappraisal* (1984), that anthrax was the culprit for the mortality, not *Yersina pestis*. One needs to be highly skeptical of Twigg's argument because it relies on what is not said in the chronicles of the plague years, primarily that no authors write about a significant number of rats, either alive or dying. The other two essays examine the social changes caused by the bubonic plague. As Cohen summarizes,

> The subsequent two chapters turn to the consequences of the plague for European civilization writ large: first, the demographic and economic consequences; second, those for the history of cultural attitudes. Again, Herlihy emphasizes that the decisive transition in the late fourteenth century from medieval to modern "systems of behavior" was not inevitable but depended directly on the most grand and horrific of external variables, the Black Death of 1348 and subsequent strikes of the disease against European populations through the early fifteenth century. (7)

Indeed Herlihy places a great deal of trust in the chroniclers' testimony in order to produce his theory that anthrax was the main culprit for the bubonic plague, and he puts a heavy emphasis on the sole effect of the bubonic plague. While I do not disagree that the bubonic plague affected the medieval sensibility, I also believe that many other social events also brought about the economic, artistic, and scientific changes from a medieval to modern period, if one actually believes that the Early Modern Period is substantially different from the medieval.

Hays's work emphasizes how epidemic diseases have influenced Western Society both on a societal and individual level. While Hays is mainly interested in post-Enlightenment medicine, he offers a comprehensive reading of numerous medieval and Early Modern diseases, including leprosy, bubonic plague, scurvy, tuberculosis, and syphilis. Hays is interested in demonstrating and explaining the ways pathological realities meet social constructions and this union is most evident in his chapter on the bubonic plague. Hays writes,

> What did medieval people make of this epidemic? In their view, what caused it? For most of those who thought about that question, divine wrath provided the most satisfactory general answer. Other causes were often cited, but for most writers such other reasons were 'secondary,' explaining how plague came in a particular time or place. Only God's wrath could

> explain such a comprehensive disaster. Furthermore, God's anger did not in this case fall on particular sinners, as was the case with leprosy. The scale of the plague suggested rather that the whole civilization, or the whole human race, was being punished. (42)

The high mortality rates and the indiscriminate nature of the disease led people to believe that the apocalypse was imminent. Certain social groups, including doctors, attempted to identify the reason for the disease in order to change the community's morality and thereby end God's wrath. And as Hays shows, once plague entered Europe, "it remained almost a constant menace for over three hundred years" (46).

Other historians have examined the primary responses of the medical community and their impact on the social community. In "Facing the Black Death: Perceptions and Reactions of University Medical Practitioners" (1994), Jon Arrizabalaga demonstrates the importance people placed in responding to the effects of the bubonic plague: "This battle was waged by *all* the people concerned with health activities: both by those educated in universities, and by those trained in the 'open' system: ordinary men and women, Jews, Muslims, and Christians—and by many who would be classified as 'quacks'" (238). Arrizabalaga notes that historians have left unexplored the record of the first responses to the plague by university-trained doctors (238). He focuses on the areas around "Italy, Provence, Languedoc, the Kingdom of France, and the Crown of Aragon" (238) and finds that:

> in opposition to the widespread historiographical view, there is no reason at all to continue separating into two different and disconnected worlds the measures against the pestilence which were established by the European civil communities and those which university physicians suggested. On the contrary, they were closely interrelated. (287)

Arrizabalaga clearly demonstrates that the civil authorities took into consideration what university-trained doctors suggested as means of preventing further infection.

While Arrizabalaga has examined the responses to the plague on the Continent, few historians have looked at the accounts of the English people in response to pestilence. However, Rosemary Horrox has recently made the study of these texts much easier. In *The Black Death* (1994), Horrox collects responses from lay, religious, and scientific people, as well as pamphlets accusing the Jews of causing the plague. I am indebted to Horrox and will be relying on her book heavily for my primary source material.

One of the most recent interdisciplinary studies of plague is Christine M. Boeckl's *Images of Plague and Pestilence: Iconography and Iconology* (2000). Boeckl examines sculpture, paintings, and drawings from the great masters of the Renaissance and Reformation. By examining these iconographical patterns, she offers a more complete picture of what it was like to live with the potential reoccurrence of plague. In some ways, I am using the same theoretical approach that Boeckl takes; however, I am examining the literary works of the fourteenth century that focus on plague.

The Origin of Plague

The bubonic plague entered Europe in October 1347, carried by a Genoese fleet returning from the Orient. The infected seamen docked in northeast Sicily in the Messina harbor. Most of the crew were either dead or dying and the Italian officials attempted to quarantine the fleet. However, lacking any knowledge about the transmission of the bacteria, the officials failed to quarantine the source of the plague. Rats and fleas scurried down the ropes of the docked ships and infected the Sicilian people within days. Plague quickly spread throughout Europe and entered southwest England through the Dorset port of Melcombe Regis in September 1348, aboard a Gascon ship (Gottfried, *Black Death*, 58). Epidemiologists estimate that primary infection killed between thirty-five to forty percent of the European population. However, plague infection did not occur once but was cyclical. As Robert Gottfried notes, "Plague would recur every few years for the rest of the fourteenth and all of the fifteenth century, and initiated an era of depopulation that would last until the sixteenth century" (*Black Death*, 130). Plague revisited England in the spring of 1361 and lasted through the winter and into spring (Gottfried, *Black Death*, 130). From 1369 to 1450, plague revisited and decimated localized areas of England (Gottfried, *Black Death*, 133).

Medieval doctors had no experience with this disease. Gottfried believes that, because of environmental changes, "the remarkably disease free" High Middle Ages brought about the needed components for pestilence (*Black Death*, 16–17). Gottfried writes, "From 1150/1200 to 1300/1350, it got colder and wetter. The Alpine glaciers in Fernau, Vernagt, Aletsch, and Grindelwald all advanced for the first time since the eighth century, with the tree line retreating in their path" (*Black Death*, 23). The colder, wetter winters combined with the encroaching glaciers created less land and resources for both humans and rats: "Archival records from livestock farmers show that the northern pastures, which had been used for hundreds of years, had to be abandoned because of the advancing glaciers and could not be used again until late in the fourteenth century" (Gottfried, *Black Death*, 23). The combination of the environmental conditions, such as the Little Ice Age, and social problems, such as overpopulation, led to the increasing possibility for plague.

The bubonic plague is caused by the bacterium called *Yersinia pestis*, and "under normal circumstances, lives in the digestive tract of fleas, particularly the rat fleas *Xenopsylla cheopis* and *Cortophylus fasciatus*, but can also live in human flea, *Pulex irritans*" (Gottfried, *Black Death*, 6). At some point, the bacilli increase and cause a blockage in the flea's digestive system (Gottfried, *Black Death*, 7). When the blockage occurs, the flea faces starvation unless it regurgitates the blockage into its host. This regurgitation pushes a high quantity of *Y. pestis* into the host which is normally lethal (Gottfried, *Black Death*, 6–7).

But the rat flea prefers rats to humans, so a second environmental step needs to occur before the human plague is created. The black rat, *Rattus rattus*, is believed to be the major carrier of infected fleas, although numerous rodents and "virtually all household and barnyard animals save the horse, whose odor apparently repels even starving blocked fleas" were secondary carriers (Gottfried, *Black Death*, 7). These secondary hosts occurred after *Y. pestis* became "enzoötic, or epidemic to a rodent population" (Gottfried, *Black Death*, 7). Known as silvatic plague, the disease kills the primary hosts first and then moves to the secondary hosts and finally to humans (Gottfried, *Black Death*, 7). The rat fleas can also "survive for between six months and a year without a rodent host in dung, an abandoned rat's nest, or even textile bales" (Gottfried, *Black Death*, 9).[14] Consequently, infected fleas could survive and transmit plague long after their primary hosts had died.

While historians and scholars refer to the pestilence that struck Europe between 1348 and 1349 as the Black Death or the bubonic plague, both references are not quite accurate. The Black Death was never used as a term in the Middle Ages. The first known reference was made by "Danish and Swedish chroniclers of the sixteenth century. 'Black' here connoted not a symptom or color but 'terrible,' 'dreadful'" (Herlihy 19). "Bubonic" is not a much better description because it implies only one type of disease, when there were actually two other variants to the disease: pneumonic and septicaemic.

Bubonic plague is the most common variant of this disease, and signs of infection occur in about six days as the bacillus has an incubation period (Gottfried, *Black Death*, 8). Gottfried writes,

> The initial symptom, a blackish, often gangrenous pustule at the point of the bite, is followed by an enlargement of the lymph node in the armpits, groin or neck, depending on the place of the flea bite. Next, subcutaneous hemorrhaging occurs causing purplish blotches and swelling in the lymphatic glands, from which bubonic plague takes its name. The hemorrhaging produces cell necrosis and intoxication of the nervous system, ultimately leading to neurological and psychological disorders. (*Black Death*, 8)

Infected people would linger in this state for a few days before death or recovery (Horrox 4). While not as lethal as other variants, bubonic plague still killed between 50 and 60 percent of those infected (Gottfried, *Black Death*, 8).

Pneumonic plague, as the name implies, is a disease of the respiratory system. More importantly, this variant enables the disease to be transmitted from human to human. Gottfried explains, "This is in part the result of pneumonic plague's peculiar etiology, for it seems to occur only when there is a sharp temperature drop and the infection moves into the lungs. After the two-to-three day incubation period, there is a rapid fall in body temperature, followed by a severe cough and consolidation in the lungs, rapid cyanosis, and the discharge of bloody sputum" (*Black Death*, 8). The sputum droplets contain the bacillus and are breathed into the lungs of the non-infected, much in the same way tuberculosis is transmitted. Death occurs in 95 to 100 percent of those infected, within a shorter period of time than bubonic (Gottfried, *Black Death*, 8 and Horrox 4).

The third variant is septicaemic, and it is the result of a massive injection of bacillus into the blood stream. Like bubonic, it is transmitted through insects, and "a rash forms within hours and death occurs within a day, before the buboes even have time to form. This type of plague is always fatal, but it is very rare" (Gottfried, *Black Death*, 8). Horrox writes, "The advantage of this explanation to historians troubled by the rapid spread of plague was that it supplied another method of person-to-person transmission by allowing a significant role to the human flea" (*Black Death*, 8). It may be possible that this variant is the one Boccaccio recalls when he writes, "How many gallant men and fair ladies and handsome youths, whom Galen, Hippocrates, Aesculapius themselves would have said were in perfect health, at noon dined with their relatives and friends, and at night supped with their ancestors in the next world!" (6). The rapid decline in health, if we take Boccaccio literally, would necessitate some variant of the plague which would kill within eight to twelve hours, and septicaemic would be that variant.

It is difficult to imagine a pestilence so virulent that it would take the life of one in every two or three people. We can only begin to imagine the emphasis placed on this disease when we compare how our society has changed since the advent of AIDS, a disease which has affected only a comparatively small fraction of the American population. Bubonic plague was read along similar moral lines as leprosy; however leprosy was not an epidemic. As time continued, medieval people realized that this was not the end of the world and certain responses to this disease could reduce infections. A slight change in interpretation led individuals to see the disease as not totally controlled by God, but also affected by human action. When syphilis entered society, the interpretation of both leprosy and bubonic plague were employed for syphilis. In this sense, syphilis was seen as a disease that was being sent to punish a specific sin in an individual, just as leprosy had been seen. However, since syphilis affected the sexual organs, it soon became evident which sin the disease punished. Consequently, the moral interpretation of the disease moved from spiritual to carnal sins; and carnal sins, like protection from the plague, are events that human beings can control.

Sexing Leprosy in the Modern Period

> Never was the influence of medicine on literature and art stronger than during the Renaissance.
>
> —Mikhail Bakhtin, *Rabelais and His World*, 360

Previously, I argued that the connection between leprosy and sex is not as prevalent in the Middle Ages as most literary critics and historians like to believe. I am not, however, arguing that the connection between leprosy and sex does not exist. Rather, it was developed and formalized in a later period because of the birth of a new disease, syphilis. Moral associations people placed on syphilis demonstrate both a new concern about sexuality and a movement from public morality to private morality.

The Origin of Syphilis

The medical relationship between leprosy and syphilis is a complicated one. In this section, I provide a summary of the debate over the origin of syphilis in order to demonstrate that at least for Early Modern Europeans, syphilis was a new disease. At that point, I demonstrate how medical doctors and laypersons approached this new disease from within the framework of learned medical traditions. Since both leprosy and syphilis make their presence known on the skin of a patient, doctors first approached syphilis along the same theoretical lines that they had approached leprosy. Therefore, syphilis acquired moral connotations commonly associated with leprosy, connotations that focused on social stability, rather than sexuality. However, as more doctors and laypersons lived through the experience of syphilis, a clear connection was made between the disease and its means of transmission. When this occurred, syphilis was considered a venereal disease. Since syphilis and leprosy were so closely linked from early on, leprosy was imbued with moral connotations earlier associated with syphilis and sexuality. The belief that leprosy reflected sexual sins existed mainly in the sixteenth and early seventeenth century, not in the Middle Ages.

One of the most heated debates in the history of diseases concerns the origin of syphilis. The central issue is whether or not syphilis was present in Europe prior to Columbus's return from the New World. On one side of this debate lies the "American" theory of syphilis, which relies heavily on literary sources and claims that no one in Europe seemed to recognize syphilis as a disease prior to Columbus's voyage. The other side argues that syphilis is part of a category of diseases known as *Treponema*; other diseases in this category are endemic syphilis, yaws, and pinta (Grmek 134). According to these theorists, the germ that creates syphilis was always present in Europe, but transformed from yaws to syphilis during the Renaissance.

In *Diseases in the Ancient Greek World*, Mirko Grmek summarizes leading medical historians' theories concerning syphilis and provides the reader with his own version. The first theorist to identify and propose that the germ *Treponema* named more than one pathogen was Ellis Herdon Hudson. Hudson proposed that *Treponema* altered its state according to climate and geography. Grmek states,

> Hudson arrives at a series of speculative conclusions: that the cradle of treponematosis was equatorial Africa, where the disease may have started in Paleolithic times with clinical manifestations almost identical to those of yaws. . . . This disease then accompanied primitive hunter-gatherers as they migrated over the African continent. With them, it crossed the Mediterranean and arrived in Europe. (135–6)

Venereal syphilis, according to Hudson, was caused by the development of urban living which started as early as 6000 B.C., and the disease existed in Greece about 900 or 800 B.C. (Grmek 136). What prevented most medical practitioners from recognizing this disease was the confusion between syphilis and leprosy. Both diseases are skin ailments, and modern historians believe that medieval doctors may have used the umbrella term "leprosy" for a host of skin diseases, including syphilis. Hudson, for instance, believes that syphilis existed in the Middle Ages; however, doctors misdiagnosed syphilis for leprosy.

In opposition to Hudson, Cecil John Hackett proposed that the four *treponema* are really "four different nosological categories" and that simple environmental change could not alter them (Grmek 137). Accordingly, Hackett suggests that ships introduced venereal syphilis throughout the Mediterranean, especially during the Roman conquest in the first century B.C. (Grmek 137). A more recent anthropologist, Don Reginald Brothwell, who proposes a later date and origin for venereal syphilis, accepts Hackett's theory. According to Brothwell, syphilis appeared in the Far East "*at least* two thousand years ago" (qtd. in Grmek 138). Grmek summarizes, "If [Brothwell] is correct, the spread of venereal syphilis from Asia into the Americas via the Pacific islands and into Europe via the expanding Arab world could not have taken place until the end of the Hellenistic period" (138).

A supporter of Hudson's hypothesis that human beings have always lived with this disease is the epidemiologist Aidan Cockburn. According to Cockburn's theory, treponemes began attaching themselves to human and animal hosts. Some of these treponemes are symbiotic and others pathogenic. Cockburn asserted that a form of yaws existed in apes and that human beings share a common ancestor, so this disease has endured since the dawn of man. However, Cockburn's theory has its difficulties. As Grmek argues, "The only form of syphilis known to exist in animals whose microbial agent has been definitely isolated is one that affects not apes but rabbits" (139). Therefore the common ancestral connection is moot. Grmek offers a way around the problem of no ancestral connection by stating that a disease transference may have occurred from rabbit to man when rabbits were domesticated (139). Thus, according to Cockburn's theory, *treponematosis* existed since the first man began to domesticate animals, and through geographic and climactic changes, the disease altered into the four forms. Eventually through the introduction of clothes, an emphasis on hygiene, and the development of certain sexual behaviors, other diseases were eliminated and venereal syphilis survived. As Grmek summarizes Cockburn's view: "The discovery of America and the pandemic of venereal syphilis are not causally related but are parallel results of one common sociocultural factor, namely, the transformation of society due to the Renaissance and the Reformation" (Grmek 139).

Mirko Grmek adds a new theory to this already complex debate. Three of the four *treponema* diseases produce marks on skeletal bones: Venereal syphilis, endemic syphilis, and pinta (Grmek 140). However, none of the bones recovered in Europe have these bone lesions. Grmek states,

> The historical and epidemiological reconstructions of Hudson, Hackett, and Cockburn are based on general biological considerations and the current distribution of four syphilitic diseases. They neglect specific historical information, and all of them face a major difficulty: the osteoarchaeology of the eastern Mediterranean. They do not take account of the fact that no trace of syphilis has been discovered on more than 25,000 skeletons and mummies from ancient Egypt and the Sudan or on several tens of thousands of prehistoric, ancient, and medieval skeletons exhumed in Europe and Asia Minor. In particular, it has not been possible to detect this disease on any bone from the Mediterranean. (139)

However, these bone lesions have been found on numerous pre-Columbian skeletons from the Americas (Grmek 140). Grmek underscores the osteoarchaeological evidence one more time: "no human remains older than 1500 and bearing sure signs of treponematosis have been found in Europe, Africa, or Asia" (140).

While this fact would seem to support the Americanist's view and refute those views of Hudson and Cockburn, Grmek argues that a compromise theory can still be presented. According to Grmek:

> The original treponematosis was, in my opinion, indeed a disease that mankind inherited from the ancestors of his species. For the initial phase, I accept Cockburn's hypothesis. But, believing as I do in the specificity of the three extant pathogenic treponemes, I suggest that the original one produced, in the Old World, a plesiomorphous branch, *Tr. pertenue*. Yaws, not pinta, is the ancient clinical manifestation of the microbial group.... In America, which [yaws] reached via the Bering land-bridge, the original germ had a different biological evolution. It bifurcated into *Tr. carateum* and *Tr. pallidum*, with the first more conservative branch confined to tropical zones,

> and the second, an apomorphous one, fit to conquer the world. Introduced from Haiti into Europe by sailors in the fifteenth century, *Tr. pallidum* spread rapidly over three continents of the Old World, producing either venereal or endemic syphilis, depending on sociocultural circumstances. (141–2)

Whether medical historians believe that syphilis was a new disease or an ever-present disease that altered in the Early Modern period, few can argue that at least for the European people of the Early Modern period, syphilis was a new disease. And since Europeans brought new diseases, such as smallpox, measles, typhus, and plague to the Native Americans, it is not inconceivable that the Native Americans repaid the Europeans' biological gifts with one of their own.[15]

Syphilis and Leprosy: An Interchange of Moral Associations

For the purposes of this section, I am not concerned about the origin of syphilis or whether medieval or Early Modern doctors misdiagnosed syphilis for leprosy. What I am concerned about is the construction of syphilis in literary texts, its connection to certain sins, and its connection to leprosy. At first syphilis is linked to sins common to the medieval construction of leprosy; however, as Early Modern authorities refined their theories, they connected syphilis to lechery, which also associates leprosy with sexual excesses. Therefore, it is the connection between syphilis and sin and the confusion between syphilis and leprosy that creates leprosy's association with lechery.

The connection between syphilis and sexual intercourse, however, took time to develop. At first, medical doctors did not deduce a direct correlation, but eventually found syphilis's main means of transmission. The word "venereal," meaning a disease transmitted through sexual intercourse, is introduced by the mid-sixteenth century and, although not conclusive, the most common citations in the *Oxford English Dictionary* are from the seventeenth century. To assume that people prior to the fifteenth century had some concept of venereal disease transmission seems erroneous.

As the previous sections demonstrate, the framework within which doctors viewed disease required a moral interpretation: the patient was responsible for his or her disease. A venereal disease is rightly named because within the word lies the connotations of "venus," love and "venial," sin. But one must remember that while we have clear associations between sex, sin, and disease, medieval doctors had no idea that microorganisms carried disease via sexual intercourse. As Amundsen argues, doctors "recommended sexual abstinence or at least moderation for their syphilitic patients, not in order to avoid spreading the disease, but owing to humoral pathology's principle of the supposedly deleterious effects of intercourse on certain categories of the ill who are undergoing certain kinds of therapy" (328). Medical doctors of the fifteenth century prescribed an avoidance of sexual intercourse because sexual activity could influence a humoral imbalance that could cause a certain disease to erupt. The major difference between modern and fifteenth-century medical thought is that for modern doctors the disease, for the most part, invades the host from outside the body. For medieval doctors, the potential for disease is on the inside, and all that was needed to bring about the illness is the necessary bodily imbalance.

When first faced with syphilis, fifteenth-century doctors connected the disease to other sins. Syphilis seems to have become epidemic around 1494 when Charles VIII, while campaigning in Italy, left his mercenaries to plunder Fornovo. After Charles withdrew his troops, some months later a Venetian doctor, Cumano, became the first chronicler of the disease. Cumano says he saw

> several men at arms or footsoldiers who, owing to the ferment of the humours, had 'pustules' on their faces and all over their bodies. These looked rather like grains of millet, and usually appeared on the outer surface of the foreskin, or on the glans, accompanied by a mild pruritis. Sometimes the first sign would be a single 'pustule' looking like a painless cyst, but the scratching provoked by the pruritis subsequently produced a gnawing ulceration. Some days later, the sufferers were driven to distraction by the pains they experienced in their arms, legs, and feet, and by an eruption of large 'pustules' (which) lasted ... for a year or more, if left untreated. (qtd. in Quétel 10)

Since syphilis usually made its first appearance on the sufferer's penis, it is simply logical that doctors would quickly connect the disease to sexuality. In the case of syphilis, the body gives accurate information about the cause of the ailment.

Even with accurate information concerning disease transmission, doctors still made the same moral associations with syphilis as were made with leprosy, owing to the notion that one skin disease is much like another. Another Venetian chronicler, Benedetto, writes:

> Through sexual contact, an ailment which is new, or at least unknown to previous doctors, the French sickness, has worked its way in from the West to this spot as I write. The entire body is so repulsive to look at and the suffering is so great especially at night, that the sickness is even more horrifying than incurable leprosy or elephantiasis, and it can be fatal. (qtd. in Quétel 10).

While relatively few cases of leprosy would have been present in Europe at this time, the disease still held traditional status as being one of the worst punishments. Benedetto clearly is aware that syphilis is a new disease, but his only comparison is to leprosy. It is associations like these that cause syphilis at first to import implications belonging to leprosy, and later to export its own specific sexual implications to leprosy.

Leprosy decreased, but it could never be removed from the cultural memory because it was so deeply ingrained in literature, theology, and medicine. By the end of the fourteenth century, leprosy infection declined in Western Europe. Evidence supporting the decline of leprosy comes from records of lazarettos that began to house the poor and plague sufferers because of available beds. Peter Richard states,

> The number of hospitals cannot be taken as a reliable indication of the prevalence of the disease. Early in the fourteenth century, when the number of foundations was at its peak, the disease was uncommon and declining. In 1344, four years before the Black Death reached England, St. Julian's hospital near St. Albans housed only two or three lepers, many fewer 'than could adequately be sustained.' Likewise, the early fourteenth-century revision of the regulations of Sherburn hospital allowed for the eventuality that there may not at any one time be a sufficient number of lepers in the diocese of Durham to fill the 65 places. When a place became vacant another leper from the diocese was to be admitted forthwith 'if there are that many lepers there,' otherwise the hospital authorities were to search further afield. (11)

After the fourteenth century, there were fewer and fewer lepers. One reason for this decline may be a symbiotic nature between leprosy and tuberculosis.

The relationship between leprosy and tuberculosis is another topic of heated discussion for scholars of nosology, but it is clear that there is some connection between these two diseases. One theory has been that leprosy and tuberculosis have a mild antagonism; when one disease is prevalent, the other disease is rare (Grmek 203). Grmek believes that this is too simple an explanation for the following reasons: some tuberculosis suffers have leprosy, tuberculosis has been uncovered in African areas of high leprosy infection, and the reduction of tuberculosis in Scandinavia did not bring about an epidemic of leprosy. Grmek states,

> These arguments effectively destroy the notion of a simple antagonism between the two diseases. But they do not, in my opinion, destroy the historical explanation for the disappearance of leprosy in medieval Europe, according to which it was the result of competition between the two related mycobacteria, with the issue depending on numerous ecological factors and the dynamics of European pathocoenosis as a whole. (203)

Grmek argues that competition between the diseases is highly complex, and part of the answer lies in the age of a person who is infected. Children tend to be more receptive to leprosy, and the first infection of tuberculosis "is closely dependent on sociocultural factors" (Grmek 204). Consequently, "a slight shift can ultimately reverse tendencies and make one disease dominate or even almost eliminate another" (204). This appears to have happened with leprosy in the fourteenth and fifteenth century, but the disease still remained in the forefront of people's minds, primarily through literary and theological transmissions of knowledge.

When syphilis made its appearance in Europe, the old traditions of leprosy came to bear on the new disease even though few doctors, priests, or authors had seen any lepers in hundreds of years. For example, the fifteenth-century Roman chronicler Sigismondo dei Conti "saw a parallel between the arrival of pox in Italy with the introduction of leprosy by Jews when they were driven out of Egypt" (Arrizabalaga, et al. 24). Also Hans Widmann of Tübingen, a medical inspector of lepers, wrote a treatise on the signs and symptoms of syphilis. Concerning this treatise, Karl Sudhoff states,

> The methods of Widmann present points of considerable interest. He has to distinguish the disease by differential diagnosis from those conditions closely allied with Leprosy. He had for long professionally occupied himself with this attempt. As a prophylactic measure he warns men to avoid, as contagious, the breath of sufferers who are afflicted with the *morbus gallicus*. When in the presence of those actually infected it is best to stand on the lee-side. This precaution had been followed for centuries in the case of lepers. (xxxviii)

What is evident from Widmann's treatise is that the medical community attempted to diagnose through association; the ideas commonly associated with leprosy were being attached to the new disease, syphilis.

The first reports of the disease made connections between syphilis and morality, but these moral associations surprisingly, at first, did not condemn sexuality. In *The Great Pox*, John Arrizabalaga, John Henderson, and Roger French state, "Only half of the sixteen earliest chroniclers mentioned the association between sexual activity and catching Mal Francese" (35). Furthermore, the Blasphemy edict, which was issued 7 August 1495 by the Emperor Maximilian, states that syphilis is a punishment for blasphemy. Maximilian states that to punish blasphemy,

> previously famine and earthquakes and pestilence and other plagues were created and still in our time, as is evident, along with these and many other and diverse plagues and punishments, especially that new and most harsh disease of mankind has arisen in our day, which is popularly called the *malum Francicum*, which never had been heard of before within human memory. (qtd. in Amundsen 312)

In his analysis, Amundsen argues that blasphemy was a more serious sin to some fifteenth-century people than was fornication (312). In the past chapter, we have seen an emphasis on the spiritual sins, particularly Envy under which blasphemy is a subset, in the literary, medical, and theological works of the Middle Ages. We will also see, when we turn to the bubonic plague, that many chroniclers believed that blasphemy or false oaths caused bubonic plague. Therefore, it would make sense that chroniclers of a new disease would use the same structure that had been applied by past medical arguments when diseases appeared *de novo*.

The first medical chroniclers of this new disease also chose sins other than fornication as the cause of syphilis. Since medicine was framed by a Christianized version of Galenism, and since moderate fornication was a part of a healthy life, fifteenth-century doctors chose to emphasize other sins that were more socially pressing. Amundsen has done a careful study of the moral associations early chroniclers attached to syphilis, and notes that early syphilographers between 1495 and 1505 did not treat syphilis as a sexual disease but as a form of humoral imbalance, thus connecting it to other diseases and their moral implications. Doctors believed syphilis to have been caused by God's anger at human sin. Coradinus Gilinus, an Italian doctor, suggested in 1497, "The Creator on high, being angered with us at this time for our impious deeds, is afflicting us with this most terrible distemper that is raging not only in Italy but throughout the whole of Christendom" (qtd. in Amundsen 327). Gilinus attributes God's wrath to the human development of military weapons and the increasing battles amongst nations (Amundsen 327). The use of weapons and war could be linked to the sins of anger and envy, two sins most commonly associated by medieval people with leprosy. Another fifteenth-century doctor, Torrella, physician to Pope Alexander VI, tells patients to "flee from anger, sorrow, and anxiety" (Amundsen 332). Sudhoff finds that Konrad Shellig of Heidelberg (c.1495) interpreted the new disease as being "characteristically mediaeval and ... was possessed of an absurd belief in the virtue and value of an utterly decayed Chivalry.... The vice upon which he especially fixed his attention was the vain use of the Divine Name" (XVIII). This view, however, is absurd only in light of modern medical accomplishments. From within the moral framework which these doctors inherited and through which they viewed disease, it made all the sense in the world.

By 1502, medical doctors were still connecting syphilis directly to sins associated with leprosy. However, doctors were beginning to focus on the sins that had some type of sexual connection. In Juan Almenar's treatise *De morbo Gallico libellus* (1502), leprosy and syphilis are clearly connected: "*spirituales medici* say that different sicknesses occur on account of different sins, such as quotidian fever on account of the sin of pride, gout on account of sloth, leprosy on account of *luxuria*, and so on concerning others. Therefore, since this disease resembles leprosy it must be attributed to *luxuria*" (qtd. in Amundsen 348). What seems to be developing by the sixteenth century are connections between leprosy, syphilis, and lechery. At some point during the sixteenth century, the cause of leprosy changed from a spiritual sin, such as envy and wrath, to a carnal sin, that of luxury or lechery. The primary cause of this change seems to be an equation of two skin diseases, leprosy and syphilis, since one disease, syphilis, is clearly sexual in nature.

The connections between syphilis, leprosy, and lechery seem to be associated with the poison damsel myth that was developed in the Middle Ages and reached its zenith at the outbreak of syphilis in the Renaissance. The first recorded articulation of the poison damsel myth as it relates to syphilis occurs with Konrad Schellig in 1497. In *Tractatus de pestilentia*, Schellig argues, "The most extreme care must be taken lest one engage in sexual intercourse with a pustulous woman, or even with a healthy woman with whom a pustulous man has lain recently, in order to avoid the risk of contagion. For already it is known by experience that one following a pustulous man is infected" (qtd. in Amundsen 323). Amundsen argues that Schellig is not simply transferring ideas about leprosy to syphilis, because Schellig states that he has experience with this means of infection. Sudhoff, on the other hand, argues that Schellig's "personal acquaintance with Syphilis was obviously of the slightest" (xxi). Many doctors stated that they had experience with procedures and even cured patients, claims we know now to be false, as Sudhoff proves by examining Schellig's later works. Schellig's lack of experience with this disease early in his career demonstrates how completely ingrained the connection between syphilis and leprosy had become. The associations common to the *mulier leprosa* were being transferred to beliefs about syphilis. Moreover, one can see a slight change in medical belief because now a pustulous woman, as well as a woman who has lain with a syphilitic, can transmit the disease to a healthy male. This association is more medically accurate for syphilis than for leprosy, but at the heart of this belief lies the poison damsel myth that began with leprosy in the Middle Ages.

While there were some changes in the poison damsel mythology when applied to syphilis, other medical doctors retain the same lines of argument that were seen with respect to leprosy, particularly the perceived immunity of women to the disease. In 1499, Petrus Pinctor, an Italian medical doctor and one of Pope Alexander VI's physicians, states that contagion of syphilis occurs through the air and around marshy places (Amundsen 342). Pinctor goes on to explain that the disease attacking Italy is "the third species of variolae, that is, *aluhmata*" (Amundsen 341). He then adds:

> This sickness is quite contagious by means of sexual intercourse with a woman who has this *morbus aluhumata* and especially one with whom a man who has this disease has had sexual intercourse. For on account of a man's warmth and the openness of the pores of the *membrum virule* the vapors, when corrupted by matter and having increased, corrupt him quite quickly. For this cause and reason, intercourse must be avoided with a woman who is suffering from *morbus aluhumata*. A woman, however, is not thus infected, unless perhaps from frequent intercourse with an infected man, since her matrix is cold and dry, dense and very little receptive to

> damage. Indeed the semen of one suffering from *aluhumata*, once it has been received by her, is quite quickly ejected or, if retained, is quickly destroyed. (qtd. in Amundsen 342–3)

The poison damsel myth, a small part of the culture of leprosy in the Middle Ages, is transferred to syphilis in the Renaissance. Once again, the woman becomes a powerful monster, who is immune to the effects of the disease but able to pass the disease onto unsuspecting men. Pinctor continues by saying that while there are authorities who "say that this happens in lepers, we, however, also assert that it occurs in those who are suffering from this disease" (qtd. in Amundsen 343).

Once syphilis became endemic, few authorities stated that the disease was not punishing individuals guilty of lechery. This moral stance seems to become so firmly established because medical doctors grasped the right means of transmission. The sinful connection, therefore, was logical. Unlike leprosy, syphilis appeared on the sexual organ; therefore, individuals guilty of lechery face the punishment of syphilis. The epidemic nature of syphilis is underscored by William Clowes's testimony that fifteen of every twenty diseased people taken to St Bartholomew's Hospital would have the pox (Williams 129). Further, Clowes's own writings about the disease demonstrate the value-laden descriptions that had passed from the Continent to England. As Clowes writes in 1579,

> The cause whereof I see non so great as the licentious and beastly filthye life of many lewd and idell persons, both men and women, about the citye of London and the great number of filthye creatures: by means of which disordered persons some other of better disposition are many tymes infected and many more lyke to be. (qtd. in Williams 128–9)

The social interpretations of this disease centered on the uncleanness and lecherous behavior of those infected. Both syphilis and leprosy are skin diseases that make their presence known on the body. When one became associated with sins of sexuality, so did the other disease. It is a simple *hic ergo hoc* formula: If leprosy and syphilis are similar skin diseases, and syphilis is understood as punishing sexual sins, then leprosy must also be punishing sexual sins.

Besides their moral, sexual, and cultural connections, leprosy and syphilis also shared one of the same saints. As Arrizabalaga and others state, "Long widespread all over Europe, the cult of St Job culminated in the sixteenth century. For several centuries Job was invoked as the patron saint by sufferers of worms, leprosy, cutaneous complaints, afflictions and melancholy" (52). By the late fifteenth century in Farrarra, Job was connected with syphilis (Arrizabalaga et al. 52). The medical, theological, and popular cultures of the Renaissance placed common interpretations that surrounded leprosy onto syphilis when it was first introduced. Literary authors also employed these parallel interpretations in the Early Modern Period. Eventually, the transference of moral beliefs about the cause of leprosy that were first placed on syphilis shifted. This shift revived and transferred sexual associations now common to syphilis back onto leprosy.

By examining the social construction of disease throughout the medieval and modern period, one sees a logical, rational attempt of people to take control of the deadly epidemics. People of the Middle Ages were fairly content in the assumption that leprosy was a disease sent by God to identify those that threatened the community through spiritual sins, because few lepers existed in the later Middle Ages and because contagion was low. When bubonic plague struck, people attempted to interpret this new disease along similar lines as that of leprosy; however, the level of infection exceeded leprosy's, and plague was more easily transmitted. Now the innocent were being punished alongside the guilty. God, in a sense, moved from being the protector of the social order to its destroyer. Eventually, human beings realized that this disease was not the end of the world, and they started to generate ideas on how to protect oneself and one's family from the ravages of bubonic plague. When syphilis struck, humans resorted to the same interpretation that they had used for leprosy and bubonic plague. With syphilis, however, a clear connection could be made between the disease and sin; consequently, syphilis was associated with the carnal sins, an act much more controllable by man. The interpretation of syphilis led to an interesting phenomena whereby leprosy was attributed to the carnal sins, because that too was a way of taking the disease out of God's hands and placing it into man's hands. Because literature participates in the same social system as medicine and theology, one can see in literary texts the same movement concerning the diseases that I have just traced. More importantly, with the moral interpretation of leprosy, bubonic plague, and syphilis clearly established, one can see the social concerns these artists struggled with in their own period. For many of the medieval authors, the spiritual sins were more dangerous than were the carnal sins. Not until the Renaissance does one see a change in literary emphasis from the spiritual to the carnal.

CHAPTER THREE

Leprosy and Spiritual Sins in Medieval Literature

In this chapter, I examine two Middle English works that seem to imply or state some relationship between leprosy and sexuality. On closer examination, only one of these works, *The Pricke of Conscience*, conveys a relationship between leprosy and lechery somewhat similar to modern definitions of a venereal disease. However, this work's connection between leprosy and lechery seems not to have taken hold in the literature of the Middle Ages, for numerous other works identify leprosy as a punishment for various spiritual sins, rather than carnal sins. The second half of this chapter examines Chaucer's Summoner, the anonymous *Amis and Amiloun*, and Robert Henryson's *Testament of Cresseid* in order to establish that leprosy was more commonly associated with spiritual sins than the carnal sins. The spiritual sins that the lepers were often supposed to have committed were sins that threatened the stability of the community. God infects people with leprosy in order to identify those who threaten the power structure of the society. The disease, therefore, is a defender of the *status quo* because it protects those already in power from being usurped by others.

The Pricke of Conscience and Gower's *Mirrour de l'omme* and *Confessio Amantis*

There are few literary works in English that either deal with or even mention leprosy. The anonymous *The Pricke of Conscience* (c.1340) and John Gower's *Mirrour de l'omme* (1376–79) are the only two extant works by popular English authors of the Middle Ages that connect leprosy to lechery. *The Pricke of Conscience*, a Northumbrian penitential poem, categorizes different types of sin. In the section "The Maladies of the Soul," the author describes how each type of ailment is connected to one of the seven deadly sins: "And som, for þe syn of lechery, / Sal haf als þe yvel of meselry" (3000–1). This extremely influential work, indicated by a large number of extant manuscripts, clearly connects leprosy to lechery. But it does not appear that the connection between leprosy and lechery took hold in the later Middle Ages, primarily because most works that mention leprosy connect the disease to other sins. *The Pricke of Conscience* also deviates from other general patterns of organization, specifically the addition of other sins to the regular seven deadly sins. As Bloomfield writes about the poem,

> The addition of sins to our concept is not unknown, but seven extra is somewhat unusual. It really cuts at the heart of the concept, for it indicates that the author or his source felt that not all particular sins could be adequately traced to the deadly seven. The lines quoted above reveal a kind of dissatisfaction with our tradition. (177)

If the author of *The Pricke of Conscience* was dissatisfied with the traditional presentation of the seven deadly sins, he may also have been dissatisfied with common associations between sin and disease. More importantly, the connection between leprosy and lechery does not necessarily mean that this disease was seen as a punishment for having sex. Rather, it was a punishment connected to the potential threat that lechery, not sex, can have for a community. Since this work deviates from a variety of general patterns found in the Middle Ages regarding both the Seven Deadly Sins and moral associations of disease, one can regard this work as either an aberration or possibly the only surviving source of a line of thought that ceased to exist.

Like the author of *The Pricke of Conscience*, John Gower also connects leprosy to lechery in his French work, *Mirrour de l'omme*. A closer examination of the connection, however, demonstrates that he is evaluating leprosy metaphorically and with an emphasis on leprosy's threat to the community, not on its venereal nature. According to Bloomfield, other English authors make connections between disease and sin, but "Gower's comparisons are the most detailed we have so far encountered in English" (196). Gower believes that lechery, like leprosy, stains the body and soul (9461–65). Secondly, like leprosy, lechery threatens the social order by making people turn from good to bad (9646–49). As Gower states,

> Lepre est auci si violente
> Que l'air ove tout le vent que vente
> D'encoste luy fait corrumpu:
> En ce Luxure represente;
> Car par tout, u q'elle est presente,
> Les gens q'a luy se sont tenu
> Leur bonnes mours et leur vertu,
> Dont l'alme serroit maintenu,
> Fait destourner en mal entente. (9649–9657)

> Second, Leprosy is so virulent that it corrupts the air together with all the wind that blows by its side, and in this respect stands for Lechery. Wherever Lechery goes, she perverts the people who hold to her, turning the good habits and virtues whereby their souls ought to be maintained into evil intent, so that they scarcely perceive their folly, for they are deceived in youth and in old age. (trans. Wilson 133)

Gower is not saying that leprosy is caused by lechery; instead, he is arguing that lechery is similar to leprosy. Both corrupt the morals of others, thereby threatening the established community. Medieval people generally believe that leprosy was a contagious disease that could be transmitted through the air. Hays speaks to the contagionist theory: "By the later Middle Ages the doctrine of contagion was more and more frequently applied to leprosy, perhaps because contagionism seemed to explain other diseases (especially plague)" (24). The breath from a leper could corrupt a person who did not have leprosy. This corruption would influence the person's morals and virtues, in much the same way leprosy influences the body's humoral system. Likewise, lechery perverts good deeds because people are simply concerned about desiring others. The connection between leprosy and lechery for Gower is metaphoric at best, very far from the causal relationship that literary critics want to see in medieval literature.

Gower's characterization of leprosy varies from one work to the next. There seems to be some connection between leprosy and lechery in the *Mirrour*, but Gower's *Confessio Amantis* uses leprosy in a non-sexual way to demonstrate how the disease works as a benefit to the community. Like theological and medical writers, medieval literary authors connected leprosy to different types of moral failings, particularly envy, anger, and avarice. The connection between envy and leprosy occurs in an understated and often overlooked aspect of Gower's *Confessio Amantis*. In reference to Gower's story of Constantine and Sylvester, Brody writes, "Although John Gower's rendering of the story in the *Confessio Amantis* (1390–1393) does not make the cause of Constantine's leprosy explicit, it does imply that the disease is punitive" (158). Brody then moves on to other analogues of this tale without returning to Gower's rendition. While it is true that Gower does not explicitly state the cause of leprosy, he does imply that the disease is caused by Constantine's envy and his separation from God.

In the story of Constantine and Sylvester, Gower introduces Constantine as "the worthy Emperour of Rome, / Suche infortunes to him come, / Whan he was in his lusti age, / The lepre cawhte in his visage" (II.3189–3191). At this point, Constantine is a pagan and is in search of a cure for his disease, relying mainly on physicians who advise him to "bathe in childres blood" (II.3206), a remedy not uncommon to medieval prescriptions. The good mothers of Rome provide Constantine with their children; however, Constantine is unable to bring himself to kill the children. Constantine thinks "how that it was noght good / To se so mochel mannes blod / Be spilt for cause of him alone" (II.3283–3285). Instead, Constantine releases the children back to their mothers and "thurgh charite thus he despendeth / His good, wherof that he amendeth / The povere people, and contrevaileth / The harm, that he hem so travaileth" (II.3311–3314). What the pagan Constantine shows is selflessness as he puts his people ahead of his personal needs.

Because of his charity, Saint Peter and Saint Paul tell him how to cure his leprosy when they visit Constantine in a dream (II.3333–3336). Constantine must visit the Christian leader Sylvester and his clergy members, all of whom Constantine "hast destruid to mochel schame" (II.3355). Sylvester teaches Constantine Christianity, and upon Constantine's taking the faith and baptism, his leprosy falls off: "lich as thei weren fishhes skales / Ther fellen from him now and eft, / Til that ther was nothing beleft / Of al his grete maladie" (II.3456–3459). Constantine is now cleansed in both body and soul, and Rome becomes a Christian city. Gower's narrator, Genius, explains the story to Amans:

> Bot forto go ther I began,
> How charite mai helpe a man
> To bothe worldes, I have said:
> And if thou have an Ere laid,
> Mi Sone, though miht understonde,
> If charite be take on honde,
> Ther folweth after mochel grace.
> Forthi, if that thou wolt pourchace
> How that thou miht Envie flee,
> Aqueinte thee with charite,
> Which is the vertu sovereine. (3497–3507)

Clearly the moral of the tale is that charity cures the sin of envy; therefore, through logical indirection, Constantine's leprosy was a punishment for his envy. Amans underscores the connection between the tale and envy when he says:

> Mi fader, I schal do my peine:
> For this ensample which ye tolde
> With al myn herte I have withholde,
> So that I schal for everemore
> Eschuie Envie wel the more. (3508–3512)

But what is not clear is what Constantine was envious of in the tale for he "[e]shuie Envie wel the more." One logical deduction is that by forgoing the use of children's blood to cure his leprosy, Constantine demonstrates that he is a servant to his people, thereby eschewing envy at least of his people. Constantine declares, "Who that woll maister be, / He mot be servant to pite" (3299–3300). In order to be a good master, Constantine learns he needs to serve, to be a servant of pity. Therefore, Constantine refuses a cure that would affect his people, and he decides to give all his treasures to the poor (3305–3310). Constantine is no longer interested in garnering wealth; instead, he gives his wealth to help his people. He forgoes envy and avarice, replacing them with pity and generosity.

Constantine's sins can only be inferred from Genius's and Amans's moralization of the tale. But many of the stories in the *Confessio Amantis* seem very loosely connected to the sin being treated. Gower sees envy as being both abominable toward God and unprofitable for man (II.3100–3110). Brody rightly states, "The story of Constantine reveals the same structure as the tale of Heinrich and indeed of most stories in which a man is first punished by and then cured of leprosy: the leprosy chastises the estrangement from God, and the submission to God brings about the cure" (159). But the cure is interestingly entangled with Constantine's relationship to his people. After choosing not to kill his community's children, Constantine then orders

> His tresour al aboute
> Departe among that povere route
> Of wommen and of children bothe,
> Whereof thei mihte hem fede and clothe
> And saufli tornen hom ayein
> Withoute lost of eny grein. (II.3305–3310)

Because of this charity, the women pray for Constantine; this prayer brings him closer to God, but his actions alone are not enough to bring about his physical cure.

Not only does Constantine need the help of his people to pray for him, but he also needs to place himself in a socially inferior position to Sylvester in order to be cured. This social positioning can be seen when Constantine asks the apparitions of Saint Paul and Saint Peter their names and estates (II.3370). The narrator tells Amans, "And thei him tolden what thei hihte, / And forth withal out of his sihte" (3371). The estate is an obvious omission by the apparitions, and relates to the stateless nature of Heaven. More importantly, the omission of Paul and Peter's estate relates to what Sylvester will teach Constantine about Christian law. As Sylvester explains to the emperor, on Judgment Day every man must face his own deeds:

> There mai no gold the Jugge plie,
> That he ne schal the sothe trie
> And setten every man upriht,
> Als wel the plowman as the knight:
> The lewed man, the grete clerk
> Schal stonde upon his oghne werk. (II.3419–2424)

Constantine has brought himself closer to God and he has shown pity and charity toward his people. Through Sylvester, Constantine is learning that he is simply a man, a man who will be judged like all other men on good deeds and faith. In order to demonstrate his learning, Constantine must place himself in a subservient position to Sylvester and to God. His subservience brings Constantine the final steps toward the healing of both his body and his soul.

Once healed, Constantine converts his city and builds two churches for Saint Paul and Saint Peter (II.3471–3479). God is then able to talk directly to the people of Rome and says, "To day is venym schad / In holi cherche of temporal, / Which medleth with the spirital" (II.3490–2). Because of Constantine's good deeds toward his people, God allows Constantine the opportunity to show his true character by becoming subservient to Sylvester and to God. This subservience allows God, through Constantine's proper ruling, to speak to the people and to improve their community. Constantine places his people above his own personal gain; therefore God rewards him both personally and professionally. While Gower does not link leprosy to a specific sin in the *Confessio*, one cannot ignore that both Amans and Genius moralize the tale of Constantine as a demonstration of envy, one of the spiritual sins. Constantine also shows that he has forsaken avarice by giving his hoarded treasure to his people. Constantine's leprosy is connected to the avarice that he cures through charity. Only by getting rid of Constantine's envy and avarice can the Roman society advance both temporally and spiritually. Prior to his cure, leprosy identified him as a moral threat, a danger to the society. Leprosy in this story remains a divine sign from God that the leper is morally weak. The role of the people is to interpret God's sign correctly and either isolate the leper or find the spiritual cure to the disease.

While *The Pricke of Conscience* uses leprosy as a punishment for lechery, other works connect sexuality to the disease minimally, or not at all. The majority of medieval works that characterize leprosy as a punishment seem to emphasis the disease's relationship to the power structures in the community. The disease is a sign of a threat to an established community, and that threat, therefore, needs to be removed. By reading leprosy through a non-sexual filter, one is able to see either the complex satire or moral didacticism that many of these authors wanted to relate to their readers. Given the devastations wrought by the plague, it's not unlikely that these authors were more concerned with the communal spiritual morality of their readers than with their private carnal morality.

Geoffrey Chaucer's Summoner

In the *General Prologue* to *The Canterbury Tales*, Chaucer demonstrates what happens when people fail to recognize signs of leprosy that God sends. Chaucer uses leprosy to demonstrate a threat to members of society, in much the same way Gower used it in the *Confessio*. The major difference, however, is that neither the community nor the leper takes action to correct the problem. The narrator describes the Summoner as having "a fyr-reed cherubynnes face / For saucefleem he was" (I.624–5). While "saucefleem" means pimpled and does not exclusively point to leprosy, the narrator adds:

> Ther nas quyk-silver, lytarge, ne brymstoon,
> Boras, ceruce, ne oille of tarte noon,
> Ne oynement that wolde clense and byte,
> That hym myghte helpen of his whelkes white,
> Nor of the knobbes sittyng on his chekes. (I.629–33)

In *Chaucer and the Mediaeval Sciences*, Walter Clyde Curry appears to be the first to recognize the narrator as describing the Summoner as having a form of leprosy. According to Curry, "the Summoner has been afflicted with a species of morphea known as *gutta rosacea*, which has already been allowed to develop into that kind of leprosy called *alopecia*" (38).

Curry uses the English priest and medical writer Andrew Boorde (1490–1549) to defend the claim that Chaucer is characterizing the Summoner as a leper. In *Introduction and Dietary*, Boorde writes: "*Gutta rosacea* are the Latin words that designate this malady; in English it is called 'a sauce fleume face,' and the symptoms are a redness about the nose and cheeks together with small pimples; it is a privy sign of leprosy" (qtd. in Curry 40). Along similar lines, Gilbertus Anglicus (d.c.1250) identifies *Gutta rosacea* as "an infection of þe nose withoutenforþ of moche reednes" (Getz 86). Gilbertus declares that this sign is "a token þat a man is disposid to be a mesel" and that the disease comes from the blood or from choler (Getz 86). If it comes from blood, "þes be þe tokenes: iching of þe nose and lyking in þe yching, and breking vp of pemples þat soone turnen to quytour" (Getz 86–7). Clearly Chaucer's narrator describes the red-faced, pimpled Summoner as the medical community describes the symptoms of leprosy. Furthermore, the cures that fail the Summoner are common to the cures described in medical manuals. For example, quicksilver, mercury, and white lead (*ceruce*) are all mentioned as cures for leprosy in *Liber de Diversis Medicinis* (c.1422).[1]

Some critics believe that the Summoner's condition more accurately reflects scabies than leprosy. Scabies is a general term for a scaly skin disease caused by a parasite and is extremely itchy. Saul Brody did not deal with Chaucer's Summoner because Brody believed the diagnosis to be questionable. Nevertheless, he sides against Curry and with Pauline Aiken, who believes that the Summoner suffers from scabies, and that Chaucer's source for this information is Vincent of Beauvais (Brody 12–3). The essential problem with differentiating between scabies, leprosy, and any number of other skin ailments is that medieval doctors often grouped different types of skin ailments together. For example, Lanfrank's *Science of Cirurgie* states that the leper will have other common signs, such as "pustulis in his tunge,

& her nailis wolen bicome greet, & þer wolen wexe scabbis abouteforþ" (197). Consequently, it would be inherently difficult for one to diagnosis the Summoner as suffering from scabies over leprosy simply because according to common medical theories, if the person was suffering from leprosy, he or she would also be suffering from scabies.

While the Summoner may indeed suffer from scabies, it is hard to ignore the similarity between Lanfrank's physical description of leprosy and Chaucer's description of the Summoner. Lanfrank states that a man is leprous when his hair begins to fall out, especially, "of her berd" (197). The narrator describes the Summoner's as having "scalled browes blake and piled berd" (I.627). Furthermore, Lanfrank describes *gutta rosacea* as a disease "þat is a passioun þat turneþ þe skyn of a mannys face out of his propur colour & makiþ þe face reed" (190). While the pustules around the nose could be scabies, they could also be what Lanfrank calls "cossi" and groups together with *gutta rosacea*: "Cossi ben litil pustulis & harde þat ben engendrid in þe face & principali aboute þe nose" (190). During the fourteenth century, the diagnosis medical doctors used for leprosy became more strict. In "Plague and Leprosy in the Middle Ages: A Paradoxical Cross-Immunity?" Stephen Ell writes, "If anything, [leprosy] was under-diagnosed, as influential figures such as John of Gaddesden in the fourteenth century counseled that no man be judged a 'leper' until his face had been destroyed" (347). Chaucer was familiar enough with Gaddesden to cite him as one of the authorities that the Doctor of Physics knows (I. 434). It is likely, therefore, that Chaucer is describing leprosy that is just surfacing on the Summoner's face, which is the new diagnostic technique being used by medieval doctors. The lack of any overt reference to leprosy allows the Summoner freedom to still hide amongst the healthy. He has not yet migrated to the kingdom of the ill, which makes him more of a threat because he can pass himself off as morally pure.

The clearest evidence that the Summoner suffers from leprosy is stated in the cures he has tried. For *cossi*, Lanfrank lists sulfur and for *gutta rosacea*, Lanfrank uses litarge and sulfur (190). None of these cures are mild, and it is Lanfrank who provides a warning to the reader that the cures for leprosy are "stronge medicyns, & þat [are of] greet perel" (197). Because of the similarities between doctor's descriptions of leprosy and Chaucer's description of the Summoner, and because the types of prescriptions mentioned by Chaucer are often used for leprosy, it seems likely that Chaucer expected the reader to conclude that the Summoner was leprous.

Besides similarities between the appearance and treatments of leprosy and the Summoner's ailment, there is also an interesting social connection between Chaucer's description and the diagnosis that appears in a thirteenth-century medical work. In the *General Prologue*, the narrator says of the Summoner, "Of his visage children were aferd" (I.628). Dated by Charles Singer and Ralph Majors to the late thirteenth century, Ashmole MS. 1398, folios 143–44, contains a description of leprosy that is similar to Chaucer's.

What is most interesting about this text is the fear a leper's appearance strikes in children. According to the author,

> Adiunguntur sanis libenter et si sanus etiam ignarus passionis eius ut pueri intueantur eos recto aspectu, timent, et turbantur facies eorum desperant et de nullo alio solicitantur. (Singer 239)

> They gladly have intercourse with the healthy, but if a healthy person who is also unacquainted with their ailment, as for example children, looks on them in the face [the children] are afraid, their faces are troubled and they despair even for that. (trans. Singer 238)

Lepers in both the thirteenth-century medical work and the description of the Summoner scare children. Clearly Chaucer is drawing on a host of common images about lepers that circulated in the Middle Ages. By reclaiming the meanings of these images, readers of Chaucer can begin to recognize his complex satire of his social community, a satire that is not related to an individual's sexuality, but rather to a community's social vigilance.

Other critics have had trouble understanding the connection between the Summoner's ailment and his sexuality. These critics have focused on the line that the Summoner is "as hoot ... and lecherous as a sparwe" (I.626). Because modern critics know that leprosy is not a venereal disease, they sometimes try to find other diseases that fit better as a sexually transmitted disease than leprosy. This leads some critics to argue that the Summoner suffers from syphilis, even if that disease does not appear to be present in fourteenth-century England. In "The Summoner's Occupational Disease," Thomas J. Garbáty finds the Summoner's disease to be syphilis, not leprosy. As Garbáty mourns, a little too exuberantly:

> It seems to me a great pity that not one student anthology or edition of Chaucer mentions the venereal origin of the Summoner's disease, a quality which the author so obviously intended the reader to recognize. Moreover, every footnote to sickness cites leprosy, or alopecia, without differentiating between Hansen's disease and the 'leprosy' of the medieval practitioners. This error has obscured the essence of the whole satire, whereas a venereal disease, whatever its name, points up, to its most consummate form, the bitter humour which Chaucer employs in this section. The face of the corrupt Summoner, watch-dog of morality, marks his own lechery. (357–8)

Garbáty approaches Chaucer's text with a desire to read lechery into a certain disease; however, when that reading does not quite fit, he assumes a modern medical framework by which to approach the disease. The bitter humor lies not in the fact that Chaucer uses a disease to characterize the Summoner's lechery, an aspect that we have seen is a side-effect not a cause of the disease, but rather that he uses a disease which symbolizes the

Summoner's moral failing in relation to simony.

The Summoner's lechery is simply a side effect of his leprosy. Lanfrank declares that men with leprosy "wilneþ myche to comme woþ wommen" (197). The thirteenth-century description of leprosy states, "Ardent plurimi eorum in coytu" (Singer "Thirteenth Century" 239).[2] As I have demonstrated, this desire to be with women is easily explained through humoral theory. The desire for sexual intercourse is used as a method of diagnosis, not condemnation, just as the pimples around the nose and hoarse voice are used in a similar fashion. Additionally, almost all medical manuals include that lepers have "mores mali," bad morals. Lepers were to be feared by people in the society because God had identified the leper as morally flawed.

The Summoner is guilty of selling the law of his society for his own personal benefit. Like the sin of Gehazi, servant to the prophet Elisha in the Old Testament, the Summoner's sin is avarice, particularly the sin of simony, the purchasing of ecclesiastical pardons or offices. According to the narrator, the Summoner "wolde suffre for a quart of wyn / A goode felawe to have his concubyn" (I.649–50). Furthermore, "And if he foond owher a good felawe, / He wolde techen him to have noon awe, / In swich caas of the ercedekenes cures/ But if a mannes soule were in his purs" (I.653–56). He allows concubinage for the payment of wine and protects people against excommunication in exchange for money. The Summoner affects his community in much the same way Gower says that Lechery damages the good. The Summoner is not only damaging the good citizens, but he is also selling services that are not his. Like Gehazi, the Summoner uses his social positioning not to serve his master, but to serve himself. While the Summoner is supposed to be monitoring the mores, both theological and civil, of his society, he chooses instead to corrupt them by selling his "blind eye" rather than his services. The narrator warns people to be wary of the Summoner's actions: "But wel I woot he lyed right in deed / Of cursyng oghte ech gilty man him drede, / For curs wol slee right as assoillyng savith / And also war hym of a *Significavit*" (I. 659–662). The Summoner has the power to curse even those who are innocent, and that curse will affect one's soul in the same way that absolution will save. Consequently, the narrator warns people to watch that the Summoner does not condemn them to excommunication or imprisonment.

What is most interesting is that the Summoner should be imprisoned because he is being identified by God as a social threat, symbolized by the beginning stages of leprosy. Therefore, Chaucer is critiquing the society that allows the Summoner to perform his social role even after God has identified him as a sinner. The question becomes who is watching the watchdog of society? Chaucer is criticizing the vigilance of those members of the ecclesiastical order above the Summoner, not the Summoner himself.

The abuse of power by people like the Summoner and Pardoner must have been commonplace in the late Middle Ages. Terrance McVeigh notes that the Summoner and the Pardoner are "two arch-simoniacs" (55). More importantly, McVeigh recognizes that Chaucer uses "physical abnormalities to symbolize this familiar ecclesiastical abuse" (55). Using Wyclif's text to connect sodomy and leprosy, McVeigh concludes, "Not merely does an analogy exist between simony and leprosy, between simony and sodomy, but an identification. The simoniac is a leper; the simoniac is a sodomist"(58). The connection between leprosy, simony, and sodomy hinges not on sexuality but on an inappropriate, unproductive act that threatens the community. Since leprosy is only divinely sent, the disease identifies those that threaten the stability of society. The relationship between leprosy and simony does demonstrate, to use Thomas Garbáty's words, Chaucer's "bitter humour" (358). But Garbáty is too limited about the source of humor: "The face of the corrupt Summoner, watch-dog of morality, marks his own lechery" (358). Leprosy not only marks his own lechery, but it also marks the lack of vigilance on the part of his supervisors. The Summoner's leprosy identifies him as an established threat to society because he is a simoniac.

Not only is the Summoner a danger to his community, but he can also do damage to the generation to come. The narrator concludes the description of the Summoner by stating, "In daunger hadde he at his owene gise / The yonge girles of the diocise, / And knew hir conseil, and was al hir heed" (I.663–5). The Summoner threatens the next generation in two very different ways. First, as medical works demonstrate, medieval people believed that leprosy could be transferred via women who had had sex with a leper. Through his close relationship with the girls of the diocese, the Summoner may infect the girls' future partners. Secondly, the Summoner is the girls' counselor and confidant, and what should be his teaching did not match his actions. The Summoner subverts the proper social order. Instead of searching out immoral people and sending them to either the ecclesiastical or secular authorities, he searches out morally good people and extorts money out of them or accepts bribes from morally bad people to avoid turning them over to the authorities. Furthermore, the Summoner has infiltrated the next generation and thereby has the ability to further corrupt the social order.

The Summoner's disease reflects his moral distance from God, a distance not dependent on his lechery, but related to the social order that he subverts through the selling of what is not rightfully his. One of the main differences, however, between the Summoner and Gehazi is that the supervisor of the Summoner is not observant enough to recognize the sign God is sending him. Unlike Elisha in the Old Testament, who immediately knows the whereabouts and actions of his servant Gehazi, the Summoner's supervisors are not as vigilant of their servant's actions. Chaucer is, therefore, not only condemning the Summoner and his actions; he is also condemning the lack of action on the part of high-ranking ecclesiastical authorities.

AMIS AND AMILOUN

Children may have had a good reason to fear lepers: their blood was believed to be a cure for leprosy. In Gower's *Confessio*, Constantine refuses to kill his subjects' children in order to cure his leprosy, and in Chaucer, the Summoner advises children improperly and thereby threatens the community. In the Middle English version of *Amis and Amiloun* (c.1330), children continue to play a role in the medieval construction of leprosy, as does the connection between leprosy and falsification. Furthermore, leprosy signifies a broken contract between God and man. The contract between God and man in *Amis and Amiloun* is similar to both the contract Constantine established with God that cures his leprosy and to the one the Summoner violates that has caused his leprosy. Most interesting in *Amis and Amiloun*, though, is that the contract between God and man is eventually superseded by a contract between men. To begin the discussion about *Amis and Amiloun*, it is necessary to provide a summary of the work.

There are numerous versions of the story, but MacEdward Leach believes that they can be placed into two categories: romance and hagiography (ix). The romance versions are written in variety of languages, including French, Latin, and English, and all these versions emphasize "the testing of [Amis's and Amiloun's] friendship to the point of child sacrifice" (Leach ix). The hagiographic versions alter "the testing of romantic friendship to an exposition of the virtues of two friends, so beloved of God and the Blessed Virgin that miracles are worked in their behalf, and so zealous in the cause of right and the Church that they are rewarded with martyrdom" (Leach ix). The present discussion focuses on the romance version, specifically the Middle English romance, *Amis and Amiloun*. *Amis and Amiloun* can be found in four manuscripts, and the *Auchinleck* manuscript is believed to date from "the second quarter of the fourteenth century, and probably not later than 1330" (Leach xc).

The story begins with the description of the two boys, Amis and Amiloun, who are born to two different Lombardy barons on the same day. The children become friends and look and act so alike that no one can tell them apart (15–20). The Duke of Lombardy takes the boys into his service when they are twelve, and the boys plight a friendship (50–157). The boys are not blood brothers, but sworn brothers. Upon turning fifteen, the boys are knighted, and the Duke makes Amis his butler and Amiloun his steward-in-hall (158–192). The chief steward becomes envious of the love that the duke and all the people have for the boys (205–210).

When Amiloun's parents die, Amiloun makes two identical cups and gives one to Amis and keeps the other (217–324). When Amiloun leaves to return to his parents' homeland, the two men re-pledge their friendship, and Amiloun warns Amis to beware of the envious steward (265–312). Amiloun returns to the land that has been bequeathed to him and marries, while Amis becomes more honored in the court of the duke (325–336). The envious steward attempts to befriend Amis, but Amis remains true to Amiloun. The steward becomes angry and looks for a way to do Amis harm (349–408). After a courtship and an argument over their different stations, both Amis and Belisaunt, the duke's daughter, pledge love to each other (421–672). The steward spies on them as they consummate their love and tells the duke of the affair (770–780).

The steward makes a formal accusation against the honor of Belisaunt, and Amis proclaims that he did not lie in her chamber (853–876). Because the servant is right and Amis is wrong, Amis goes to Amiloun for help (949–972). Amiloun chooses to take the fight for Amis and on behalf of Belisaunt by impersonating Amis (1105–1128). Amis and Amiloun switch places, and Amis stays with Amiloun's wife, each night feigning a strange illness that makes his body sore and placing a sword between him and Amiloun's wife as a means of separation (1129–1188). As Amiloun rides into the duke's court pretending to be Amis, a voice from Heaven tells Amiloun that if he goes through with this falsification, he will be a leper in a year (1249–1272). Nevertheless Amiloun defends his friend and puts down the steward, and the duke gives Amiloun his daughter (1369–1392). The two friends switch places again (1417–1440). Amis is married to Belisaunt, and as Amiloun goes to bed, his wife asks him where his sword is, thereby proving Amis's faithfulness to Amiloun (1453–1524). Amiloun tells the entire story to his wife who angrily berates him for his actions (1489–1500).

When two years pass, Amis and Belisaunt are now the duke and duchess, and Amiloun is a leper who has been deserted by his wife (1525–1560). Eventually Amiloun is placed in an outside hut and served by his nephew Amoraunt who swears to serve Amiloun until his death (1621–1644). By the end of the year, no more food is being given to them, so Amiloun and Amoraunt beg for food, but in the fourth year a famine makes food so scarce that the two have to travel further to find donations (1656–1860). They travel to Amis's kingdom, where Amoraunt purchases a pushcart in which he places Amiloun (1849–1872). Amiloun orders Amoraunt to tell no one who he is (1873–1874). While begging in the streets, a knight notices the dedication of Amoraunt to this leper and offers Amoraunt a courtly job, which Amoraunt refuses (1909–1944). The knight, intrigued by this refusal, tells the story in the court of Amis (1945–1992). Astounded by this tale, Amis decides that the servant must be rewarded for his faithfulness (1993–2004). Upon Amis's orders, a squire goes to take Amis's cup of wine to the leper, but when the squire arrives, the leper has the same cup (2005–2027). The squire returns to Amis and tells him about the similar cups (2029–2052). Thinking this leper has hurt Amiloun, Amis threatens to kill the leper only to find out that the leper is Amiloun (2053–2088).

Amiloun is immediately brought into Amis's castle, and both Amis and Belisaunt care for Amiloun for a year until one night an angel tells Amis in a dream that he can heal Amiloun's illness by bathing Amiloun in the blood of Amis's children (2089–2243). On Christmas Eve, Amis, with the household empty save for his children, steals into the nursery and slits all the children's throats and collects the blood (2245–2317). When Amis gives his children's blood to Amiloun, Amiloun weeps, and when Amis tells Belisaunt what he has done, she says that he has done the right action because children are numerous, but they only have one Amiloun (2318–2400). When Amis and Belisaunt go to Amiloun, they find his leprosy cured, and when they go into the nursery, they find their children unhurt and playing (2401–2424). Amiloun returns to his land with Amis, where they find Amiloun's wife about to marry a baron (2425–2458). After winning the victory against the baron and after imprisoning his unfaithful wife in a small hut to be fed only bread and water, Amiloun gives his entire land to Amoraunt and returns with Amis to Lombardy where the two eventually die on the same day and are buried together (2461–2507).

The Middle English version has many unique features, one of which is the Christianization of certain aspects of the story. In "The Middle English *Amis and Amiloun*: Chivalric Romance or Secular Hagiography?" Ojars Kratins describes the unique way this adaptation handles divine punishment. According to Kratins:

> In the Anglo-Norman versions as in all others where the motif of the warning voice appears (the *chanson de geste*, the miracle play), it comes at the point where Amiloun is about to commit technical bigamy by marrying the duke's daughter in his friend's stead. (In the Middle English poem, the friends exchange roles again before the marriage.) By transposing the warning to a spot before the combat, the English adapter provides a sound reason for Amiloun's illness and thus links the two sacrifices constituting the test of *trewþe* in the strongest possible way. (350)

Amiloun's punishment of leprosy is sound because leprosy signifies those who are guilty of falsifying their words. Because Kratins is mainly interested in a genre study, he glides over an in-depth study of the signification of leprosy in the Middle English poem, choosing instead to simply mention the Old Testament's connection between leprosy and sin. Kratins, nevertheless, identifies an important point about the story and the disease: "the English poem is no different from that in the *Vita*: it is a visitation of divine grace with the goal of verifying, before the tale is over, that both friends in the severest of trials 'trewe weren in al þing,' as the poem states at the outset" (351). Kratins also notes that this romance provides a different definition of being true, for in the tale, truth relates to man-to-man relationships, not man-to-God relationships (354). However, I disagree with Kratins's assessment that the voice's threat of the disease "is morally neutral" (350). Rather it fits common medieval beliefs about what leprosy represents.

When Amiloun, pretending to be Amis, walks into the castle to defend Belisaunt's honor, he hears a voice "fram heuen adoun" (1250). The voice declares:

> Þou kniȝt, sir Amiloun,
> God, þat suffred passioun,
> Sent þe bode bi me;

ȝif þou þis bataile vnderfong,
Þou schalt haue an euentour strong
Wiþ-in þis ȝere þre;
& or þis þre ȝere ben al gon,
Fouler mesel nas neuer non
In þe world, þan þou schal be! (1252–1260)

The voice makes it clear that leprosy will be the punishment for Amiloun's actions of falsifying his identity. If Amiloun enters the battle, within the year God will strike him down with leprosy more foul than anyone has ever seen. Not only will God punish Amiloun with a disease, but also, the voice tells him, his "wiif & alle þe kinne/ Schul fle þe stede þatow art inne, / & forsake þe ichon" (1270–2). If Amiloun is disobedient to God and violates His wishes, then Amiloun loses his entire social community through the advent of leprosy.

Amiloun clearly understands the ramifications of his actions: "Þat kniȝt gan houe stille so ston / & herd þo wordes euerichon, / Þat wer so gret & grille" (1273–75). He also realizes that he has choices, even as he is just about to enter the castle: "He nist what him was best to don, / To flen, oþer to fiȝting gon, / In hert him liked ille" (1276–78). Finally, Amiloun comes to a decision that underscores the importance he places on this man-to-man relationship, which is more important than his relationship with God:

ȝif y beknowe mi name,
Þan schal mi broþer go to schame,
Wiþ sorwe þai schul him spille.
Certes . . . for drede of care
To hold mi treuþe schal y nouȝt spare,
Lete god don alle his wille. (1279–84)

If Amiloun does not fight in Amis's place, Amis will be shamed because the people will find out that Amis was with Belisaunt. However, if he does fight, he will be shamed because he will contract a disease that represents his disobedience to God.

In other versions of the story, the punishment is petrification, not leprosy. Leach explains, "Leprosy was chosen as a substitute for petrification because the bath in the blood of children was the recognized specific for it, and the author had to retain the incident of the killing of the children to be the supreme test of friendship between the two brothers. In other words, by the substitution of leprosy for petrification both the punishment and the cure become rationalized" (lxii). Leprosy also makes more sense because the disease signifies falseness. More important, the English version of this story is the only one that moves the threat of leprosy to just prior to Amiloun's falsification. In the French versions of the story, the voice announces the ramifications of Amiloun's actions when he is about to wed Belisaunt, thus being guilty of either bigamy or falsification. However, by changing the place where Amiloun is warned and by changing the moment when they resume their real identities, the author clarifies that Amiloun is punished with leprosy for the sin of falsification. Amiloun chooses to have himself shamed rather than his friend. Amiloun is more concerned with his allegiance to man than his allegiance to God. Therefore, God sends down a disease that symbolizes the falsification Amiloun has displayed.

The romance of Amis and Amiloun and the construction of leprosy in the Middle Ages highlight one aspect of the changing social relations in the late fourteenth century. In his work on the social environment in Chaucer's work, Paul Strohm argues, "Noticeable in social relations among the later fourteenth-century gentry is a partial redirection of personal loyalty, from vertical commitment to a single lord in a hierarchical system to a more horizontal dispersal of loyalties among the members of one's social group" (21). For Strohm, the gentry composes "a fourth-estate or middle grouping embracing knights, esquires, other gentle-persons, merchants, citizens and burgesses, and some other prosperous guildsmen" (11). It is within this gentry class that relationships are beginning to change, primarily in relation to how "homage and fealty [are] performed" (Strohm 15). Strohm writes,

> Old relations of vassalage based on land tenure were extensively redefined, opening the way to more flexible forms of service and more varied remuneration: sacral, sworn bonds were replaced by voluntary agreements; permanent loyalties gave way to more temporary arrangements; vertical ties of domination and subordination—while by no means wholly superseded—were everywhere set in competition with lateral ties among people in similar social situations. (1)

Amiloun demonstrates this new type of voluntary, sworn brotherhood with Amis, a person of similar social rank, both being knights, part of Strohm's fourth-estate. More importantly, the text demonstrates that the old models of homage and fealty to a superior are being modified in light of relationships bound by one's word to social equals. This fidelity to words is evident through Amiloun's acceptance of God's will to punish him with leprosy for his disobedience, rather than allow his sworn brother to face similar shame.

Leprosy is not only a punishment in this text; it also has the potential to generate rebirth by cleansing individuals and society. Amiloun's wife and neighbors have the potential to demonstrate Christian charity toward Amiloun; however, each chooses to punish the leper rather than offer comfort. After Amiloun contracts leprosy, his wife declares,

> Þou wreche chaitif,
> Wiþ wrong þe steward les his liif,
> & þat is on þe ene;

Þer-fore, by Seyn Denis of Fraunce
Þe is bitid þis hard chaunce,
Dapet who þe bimene! (1564–9).

Amiloun's wife does not understand that the reason for Amiloun's condition is not that he killed the steward but that he disobeyed God's word. Instead of comforting and caring for Amiloun, Amiloun's wife turns him out of his house. Consequently, the narrator refers to his wife as "wicked & schrewed" (1561).

Amiloun is also rejected from his place of lodging in the town. After six months of living in board, the lady of the house complains,

In þis lond springeþ þis word,
Y fede a mesel at mi bord,
He is so foule a þing,
It is gret spite to al mi kende,
He schal no more sitt me so hende,
Bi Ihesus, heuen king! (1590–6)

Instead of taking the leper in and showing him Christian charity, the lady is more concerned about her shame and chooses to throw him out. Ironically, she uses Christ's name in vain, also demonstrative of her failure to follow Christian law. Amiloun's disease allows him to see the true nature of his wife and his neighbors, a nature lacking charity and failing to follow Christian rules.

In contrast to Amiloun's wife and town are Amiloun's nephew Amoraunt and Amis's wife. Amoraunt faithfully serves Amiloun throughout the tale. Because of this faithful service, Amis gives charitably to both the leper and his servant. Amis orders his squire:

Take . . . mi coupe of gold,
As ful of wine astow miȝt hold,
In þine hondes tvain,
& bere it to þe castel-ȝate,
A lazer þou schalt find þerate
Liggeand in a wain.
Bid him, for þe loue of Seyn Martin,
He and his page drink þis win
& bring me þe coupe ogain. (2008–16)

The wine foreshadows the blood of Amis's children whom he will have to slay in order to cure Amiloun of his leprosy as well as the obvious connection to the blood of Christ shed to cleanse Original Sin. Unlike Amiloun's court, in which Amiloun was rebuked, Amis's court accepts lepers and offers them charity. Amis also calls on Saint Martin who was known to take care of lepers: "Martin was a man of deep humility. In Paris he once came face to face with a leper from whom all shrank in horror, but Martin kissed him and blessed him, and he was cured" (Ryan 295). Amis calls on Saint Martin because like Saint Martin, Amis is not repulsed by the idea of a leper; instead he treats the leper with kindness.

Amis is not the only one to receive Amiloun with love and affection. When Amiloun's identity is revealed to Belisaunt, she "aswon to grounde" (2170). The narrator further describes the scene:

As foule a lazer as he was,
Þe leuedi kist him in þat plas,
For noþing wold sche spare,
To liue in sorwe & care.
Into her chaumber she gan him lede
& kest of al his pouer wede
& baþed his bodi al bare,
& to a bedde swiþe him brouȝt
Wiþ cloþes riche & wele ywrouȝt;
Ful bliþe of him þai ware. (2173–84)

Clearly, Belisaunt demonstrates true Christian charity toward her husband's brother, a fidelity that neither Amiloun's wife or town attempted. Amiloun continues to live with them a year and the narrator declares that both husband and wife were "trewe" and "kinde" (2186). More importantly, Amiloun is denied nothing (2187–8). Consequently, when Amis tells Belisaunt that he has killed their children, she responds by saying, "God may send ous childer mo," but they have only one Amiloun (2393–96).

While it may seem that this sentiment is unrealistic and unacceptable, Belisaunt's response points to the increasing value placed on one's honor and word. Belisaunt, unlike Amiloun's wife, realizes the extent of the bond between Amis and Amiloun. While Amiloun has proven his truth to Amis, now Amis must demonstrate his worthiness in this bond by performing an equally great sacrifice. Parallel to God's sacrifice of Christ or Abraham's sacrifice of Isaac, Amis is given the choice to slay his children so that their blood will alleviate Amiloun's sin or to let Amiloun continue to suffer from leprosy. Further, like Christ, the children are resurrected.

After Amiloun is cured with the blood of Amis's children and after Amis and Belisaunt find the children unharmed, Amis and Amiloun ride out to correct Amiloun's wife:

He wolde hoom to his contray,
To speke with his wyf þat tyde;
And for she halþ his so at nede,
Wel he þouȝt to quyte hur mede. (2431–35)

Amiloun's correction relates primarily to his wife's failure to keep her word to help him in his need. Her impending betrothal to a wealthy baron is interrupted by Amiloun, and the narrator comments, "Þan wox þe lady blew and wan, / Þer was mony a sory man, / Boþ ȝong and olde" (2458–60). The community that cast Amiloun out on account of his disease remains unprosperous and melancholy. Nevertheless, the baron and his knights fight Amis and Amiloun and are eventually put down by the two friends. Amiloun punishes his wife by building her a small hut and ordering her to eat only bread and water for the rest of her life (2476–81). This action could be seen as a metaphoric leprosy instituted by man rather than God, because Amiloun removes his wife from society and gives her the board he was fed as a leper. Leprosy is divinely sent to either identify falsifiers or test the community's response. In this case, Amiloun's illness was sent as a test that the town's people failed. Thus, the leper who often represents sin and falsehood was indirectly testing the town's people to discover that they were the true falsifiers. While they did identify and remove the leper from society, they were not hospitable and true to him. Their pledged fidelity was untrue. Because Amiloun's wife was untrue to him and did not take care of him, he places her outside the community. Furthermore, those who have served him well are rewarded, such as Amoraunt who is given Amiloun's land as a reward for his tireless service (2489).

The story of *Amis and Amiloun* reflects both God's commitment to man and man's social relationship with other men. In this text, leprosy remains a divine punishment for violating one of the spiritual sins. However, God's punishment is also a test for those individuals who surround the leper. Rejected by his wife and community, Amiloun finds loyalty from his servant and, eventually, from his sworn brother, Amis. Amis sacrifices his own children in order to cure Amiloun's leprosy. God rewards this sacrificial act, and He cures Amiloun's leprosy and revives Amis's children. What God has tested is the bond between the two men, not the bond between man and God.

Interestingly, Amiloun and Amis punish Amiloun's wife along the same theoretical lines that God uses for lepers. When a person breaks his bond with God, God sends leprosy as a punishment. Other people are supposed to recognize the disease and separate the leper from society. In the case of Amis and Amiloun, Amiloun's wife breaks her word to Amiloun, specifically the marriage vow, and is punished by Amis and Amiloun by being removed from the society. By locking Amiloun's wife away, Amis and Amiloun make her into a kind of leper. Leprosy remains a divinely sent disease; however, the isolation from society becomes a punishment for breaking vows between human beings. Thus, Amis and Amiloun demonstrate proper social supervision of their community. They remove those that are false in order to protect the community. They do what the pilgrims of *The Canterbury Tales* fail to do: they recognize sinful behavior and take action before that person ruins the community.

Robert Henryson's *Testament of Cresseid*

Like *Amis and Amiloun*, which uses leprosy as a test in order to signify those who are false, Robert Henryson's *Testament of Cresseid* (late fifteenth century) also uses leprosy as a punishment for falsification. This poem in particular has suffered the most from the misinterpretation of the meaning of leprosy. Peter Richards represents the most common misinterpretation of the *Testament*: "Medieval sermons and literature, in harmony with the contemporary image of the disease, portrayed leprosy as a punishment meted out for moral failing, especially for loose, wanton, and lustful living" (6). Because literary critics connect leprosy to uncontrolled sexuality, their interpretations of the *Testament* twist both the literary evidence and historical facts to make their theory fit the text. For example, Beryl Rowland writes that "[August] Hirsch subsequently contended that medieval leprosy, widely held to originate 'ex coitu cum foeda muliere,' could be synonymous with syphilis, and modern medicine demonstrates that many conspicuous symptoms in leprosy may also be found in syphilis, a disease regarded as a great imitator" (175). Rowland concludes: "It seems possible that Fracastoro and Henryson may have been describing the same disease. If so, in giving his heroine such a savage punishment, Henryson may have been governed by a desire for realism rather than by a concern for morality" (177). Even if the disease Henryson describes were syphilis, it would still have a moral connotation, as it does in Fracastoro's work. However, as Kathryn Hume explains,

> It seems improbable that Henryson could have known about syphilis as distinct from leprosy when he wrote the poem, which is generally thought to have been composed between 1470 and 1492; and Professor Rowland herself seems to accept these dates. Whether syphilis existed in Europe at this time is hotly disputed. Some historians hold that it was brought back from the New World; others claim that it was indigenous to Europe, but had long lain dormant or been mistaken for other diseases, such as leprosy. Whichever hypothesis is correct need not concern us here, since *syphilis was not diagnosed as a separate disease* until 1493 (in Spain), and did not become at all widely known until 1495 at the siege of Naples. It did not achieve formal recognition in Scotland until 1497. Consequently, unless Henryson wrote his poem much later than has hitherto been thought, *he could not knowingly have afflicted Cresseid with syphilis*, even though its symptoms tally with hers. (243; emphasis in original)

While Hume is accurate in her rejection of the likelihood that Cresseid's disease is really syphilis supported primarily by Henryson's use of the word "leper" which makes misinterpretation rather difficult, she makes a crucial error by assuming that Cresseid's disease is transmitted sexually. Hume states, "Leprosy ... does make a positive artistic contribution to Cresseid's fall. (1) It is at least as appropriate and 'realistic' as syphilis, for ... it was widely held to be transmitted venereally. (2) Cresseid's punishment is inflicted directly by the gods" (245). There are some problems in Hume's facts and logic. First, as we have seen medieval doctors suggest that the transmission of leprosy sexually occurs with women who have had sex with lepers and then transmit the disease to healthy men. Chaucer's Summoner is an example of how a leper could infect numerous women if given the opportunity. There is no mention of or allusion to a leprous man in Henryson's work. Secondly, Cresseid is a follower of the gods Venus and Cupid. These two gods would not punish Cresseid for her promiscuity; indeed she would be praised and elevated for promiscuity in their temples. Instead, Cresseid is being punished with leprosy because her words are disrespectful and blasphemous; therefore she is guilty of spiritual, not carnal sins.

In the poem, Cresseid does not go into Venus's temple to make a sacrifice to the gods (116). Instead she goes into a "secreit orature" to "weip hir wofull desteny" (120–1). In this place, the narrator explains that Cresseid angrily calls out against Cupid and Venus (124). Not only is she angry with Cupid, but her own words demonstrate that she also lacks devotion to the gods. Cresseid states:

> Allace, that euer I maid ȝow sacrifice!
> ȝe gaue me anis ane deuine reponsaill
> That I suld be the flour of luif in Troy;
> Now am I maid an vnworthie outwaill,
> And all in cair translatit is my joy.
> Quha sall me gyde? Quha sall me now conuoy,
> Sen I fra Diomeid and nobill Troylus
> Am clene exludit, as abject odious?
>
> O fals Cupide, is nane to wyte bot thow
> And thy mother, of lufe the blinde goddes!
> ȝe causit me alwayis vnderstand trow
> The seid of lufe was sawin in my face,
> And ay grew grene throw ȝour supplie and grace.
> Bot now, allace, that seid with froist is slane,
> And I fra luifferis left, and all forlane. (126–140)

Cresseid's sin is her inability to both recognize what Cupid and Venus have done for her and to accept her role in the events of her life. She falsely accuses Cupid and Venus when Cresseid herself must accept responsibility for her actions with Troilus and Diomede. Cresseid's extended plant metaphor provides an interesting allusion to the lives of lepers and the powers of the gods. According to Cresseid, Cupid sowed the seed of love into her face and through his grace it grew; however, Cresseid's "fall" has come and the frost has left her abandoned. Cupid, however, is not done sowing. Because of Cresseid's actions, Cupid demonstrates that he can also sow the seeds of exclusion in her face by giving her leprosy, a disease which symbolizes both her falseness to the gods and her death in the material world.

Cupid's punishment of Cresseid clearly outlines her falsehood and blasphemy. After Cresseid falls asleep, Cupid appears and calls the planetary gods to descend from the spheres (146–7). When the narrator comes to Venus, he declares that she is there to defend her son's "querrell" and "mak / Hir awin complaint" against Cresseid (219–220). Cupid explains the reason for their gathering: "quha will blaspheme the name / Of his awin god, outher in word or deid, / To all goddis he dois baith lak and schame, / And suld haue bitter panis to his meid" (274–77). Cupid's accusation of Cresseid's sin focuses on her blasphemy against him and his mother, and this accusation demonstrates that Cresseid lacks the humility necessary for interactions with the gods. Her injury to the gods is similar to that of Miriam who believed that she was on the same level as Moses and lacked the humility to realize her social positioning.

Cupid also identifies that Cresseid has not taken proper responsibilities for her actions and for her social problems. Cupid defends himself and Venus:

> Saying of hir greit infelicitie
> I was the caus, and my mother Venus,
> Ane bline goddes hir cald that micht not se,
> With sclander and defame iniurious.
> Thus her leuing vnclene and lecherous
> Scho wald retorte in me and my mother. (281–6)

Cupid's argument is not that Cresseid lives an unclean and lecherous life and needs to be punished for that life. Instead, Cresseid needs to be punished for the slander and defamation she has caused both gods because they are not at fault for her social position; Cresseid is at fault. Her lechery is simply a further indictment of questionable moral character. The blame that Cresseid places on the gods for her life's injuries extends beyond Cupid and Venus to all "participants of deuyne sapience" (289). All the gods agree to take revenge on Cresseid because she is a falsifier and because she blames others for her actions; therefore the gods' revenge will be a disease that identifies her as a falsifier and a threat to others in the society.

While leprosy is always a disease divinely sent in fifteenth-century literature, Henryson's description of the making of this disease clearly follows common medical beliefs. When Saturn touches the head of Cresseid, he says,

> I change thy mirth into melancholy,
> Quhilk is the mother of all pensiuenes;
> Thy moisture and thy heit in cald and dry;
> Thyne insolence, thy play and wantones,

> To greit diseis; thy pomp and thy riches
> In mortall neid; and greit penuritie
> Thow suffer sall, and as ane beggar die. (316–322)

As demonstrated above, medical authorities believed that leprosy was caused by corrupted melancholy. Saturn turns the blood or mirth into melancholy, thereby causing Cresseid's leprosy. Similarly, Saturn changes Cresseid's temperature balance from moist and hot to cold and dry. Finally, Cresseid receives this disease because of her insolence against the gods. The other nouns, play and wantonness, are not sins, especially for a pagan god, but are the good things Cresseid was given in life. Even Cresseid recognizes the reason for her disease: "My blaspheming now haue I bocht full deir ... allace, this wofull tyde / Quhen I began with my goddis for to chyde" (354).

Because leprosy symbolizes Cresseid's falsehood toward the gods, her final complaint to lovers fits thematically better than if leprosy symbolized uncontrolled sexuality. Cresseid admonishes lovers to be truthful, rather than false as she was:

> Because I knaw the greit vnstabilnes,
> Brukkill as glas, into my self, I say—
> Traisting in vther als greit vnfaithfulnes,
> Als vnconstant, and als vntrew of fay—
> Thocht sum be trew, I wait richt few ar thay;
> Quha findis treuth, lat him his lady ruse;
> Nane but my self as now I will accuse. (568–574)

Cresseid has learned that few people are true and her leprosy represents her own falsehood. More importantly, Cresseid knows that she is the only one to blame for her condition. The narrator underscores this moral when he tells "worthie women:" "Ming not ȝour lufe with fals deceptioun: / Beir in ȝour mynd this sore conclusioun / Of fair Cresseid" (613–15). The narrator is referring both to Cresseid's untruthfulness to Troylus and to the gods. But it is the "fals deceptioun" toward the gods that brings about her leprosy.

It would appear that medieval authors connected a great number of sins to leprosy. By reducing the number of sins to just one, lechery, critics fail to take into account the varied meanings medieval authors have tried to express. While two authors appear to connect leprosy to lechery in the Middle Ages, a greater number of authors—medical, theological, and literary—seem to believe that leprosy is a punishment from God sent down to warn society that falsifiers threaten the community. These falsifiers need to be identified and removed in order for the *status quo* to remain. The sins of the guilty vary from simony in the case of the Summoner to blasphemy in *The Testament of Cresseid*. In the romance *Amis and Amiloun*, leprosy is used as a means to test the community's faith and resolve, and it tests the oaths made man-to-man rather than God-to-man. The importance placed on oaths between men demonstrates a changing society in which horizontal market relations are replacing vertical feudal allegiance.

The information authors used regarding leprosy in the Middle Ages also fits into the beliefs of the medical and theological communities. All three groups—authors, doctors, and priests—believed that leprosy was divinely sent for sins and that individuals needed to be removed for the protection of the established society. The doctor's humoral reasons for the disease did not preclude divine origin or control. Too many critics and historians want to see the medical establishment of the Middle Ages as immune from the common beliefs of the community. Doctors of the Middle Ages were an intricate and interrelated part of society and, therefore, saw the disease through the same socially constructed glasses as their social counterparts. In our own time, it is commonly assumed that most diseases come from viruses or bacteria, yet numerous people, both in the medical community and outside, declared, at first, that AIDS was a punishment sent by God for hedonistic living. Knowing how the mechanism of disease works does not always answer why a disease is created.

The first human response to an epidemic seems to be apocalyptic, as with AIDS. When bubonic plague struck Europe, people of the Middle Ages applied the same moral associations that they had used with leprosy to bubonic plague. Thus, God was punishing them for their spiritual sins. Like leprosy, bubonic plague's potential list of sins varies; however, it is much different from leprosy because plague is acute and affects large numbers of people, whereas leprosy is chronic and infects limited numbers. The large number of infections gave God total control over the disease, because no human being could figure out what sin this disease was isolating and when would God stop punishing. In other words, God moves from defender and protector of the social power structure with leprosy to one of a destroyer who seeks to end all human life through plague. But eventually human beings realize that the plague is not ending all of human civilization and that there are ways to survive the plague's mortality. In the next chapter, I explore the ways literary, medical, and theological works written around the time of plague use the same moral associations that were previously used by leprosy to explain the reason for God's wrath. These moral associations highlight what people believed were the major social problems of the late Middle Ages.

CHAPTER FOUR

Plague as Apocalypse in Medieval Literature

Leprosy and plague are often placed together as the two major diseases affecting the Middle Ages. Historians see these diseases as competitive, owing to the belief that the presence of bubonic plague in Europe further reduced the number of lepers (Hays 24). These diseases also point to a human desire to control the effects of God. Leprosy and bubonic plague are different diseases; the former is chronic and difficult to contract, while the latter is acute and easier to transmit. Leprosy allowed humans to moralize about the sins that brought about the disease, because the disease was localized and hard to contract; therefore, the moral interpretations held because there was little evidence to refute those interpretations. When bubonic plague struck, people attempted to interpret the disease along similar moral guidelines as they did for leprosy. In this chapter, I explore the different moral meanings literary, medical, and theological authors ascribed to plague. Through an examination of William Langland's *Piers Plowman*, Geoffrey Chaucer's the *Pardoner's Tale*, and the York Cycle's *Moses and Pharaoh*, I demonstrate that the authors focused on spiritual sins as the reason for the presence of plague and that these moral associations point to perceived social problems within medieval English society.

WILLIAM LANGLAND'S *PIERS PLOWMAN*

William Langland composed the variations of *Piers Plowman* between the 1360s and 1388, which means that he witnessed some of the worst mortality caused by bubonic plague. Just as plague affected his society, so does plague affect his literary characters. In both Passus VIII and XXII of the C-text, Langland provides us with the central relationship between sin and plague. Plague symbolizes and corrects a morally corrupt society. Langland employs plague whenever the characters reach a moral impasse. In Passus VIII, Piers pleads for Hunger to attack the fair field of folk because they will not work.

After Hunger attacks and the workers repent, the narrator prophesies that if the workers do not labor, Hunger will come again and through "pruyde and pestilence shal moche peple feche" (349).[1] Only after many people have died "shal deth withdrawe and derth be iustice" (352). For Langland, pestilence corrects the sinful nature of the society—in this case, a society that fails to work. But Langland uses the reference to pestilence only as a warning, as a dénouement to Hunger's attack on the fair field of folk. Only when his characters fail to heed Hunger's warning does the prophesy comes true.

The relationship between pestilence and sin climaxes in Passus XXII when the Antichrist appears and turns Truth "vp-so-down" (54). He leads many people to sin and eventually attacks Conscience with the Pride of Life, "a lorde þat lyueth after likyng of body" (71). Conscience asks Nature to defend against this attack. Nature answers Conscience's call and "cam oute of the planets / And sente forth his forreours, feuers and fluxes" (80–1). Nature's foragers, or helpers, are fevers and fluxes. Then, Old Age claims the banner of death and joins Nature creating "many kyne sores, / As pokkes and pestilences, and moche peple shente" (97–8). Nature's sicknesses spare no one: "lered ne lewed he lefte no man stande" (102). Only when man makes amends and "leue pruyde priueyliche and be parfyt cristene" (108) does Nature cease and desist. Once again, Langland employs pestilence in order to correct the sinfulness of his literary characters. Since pestilence was common during Langland's time, is it possible to read this work as a prophetic warning designed to correct the behaviors of sinful people and, in turn, alleviate God's punishment? In order to answer this question, we must first examine how much of Langland's information about plague comes from contemporary authorities, especially medical and theological authorities.

As we have seen, Langland associates plague primarily with the sin of pride. These connections between pride and plague can be found in the theological community. In 1348, John Stratford, the Archbishop of Canterbury, in a letter to the Bishop of London writes,

> [God] often allows plagues, miserable famines, conflicts, wars, and other forms of suffering to arise, and uses them to terrify and torment men and so drive out their sins. And thus, indeed, the realm of England, because of the growing pride and corruption of its subjects, and their numberless sins, has on many occasions stood desolate and afflicted by the burdens of the wars which are exhausting and devouring the wealth of the kingdom, and by many other miseries. And it is now to be feared that the same kingdom is to be oppressed by the pestilences and wretched mortalities of men which have flared. (Horrox 113–14)

Evidently, the Archbishop believed that England was not going to be spared God's anger. More importantly, while many sins are mentioned, the only one clearly established is that of Pride, a sin Langland will return to over and over again.

Langland's beliefs about the origin of plague can be interpreted on both a moral and natural level. The clearest definition Langland offers of pestilence occurs in Passus V:

> Resoun reuerentliche tofore al þe reume prechede,
> And preuede þat this pestelences was for puyre synne
> And the south-weste wynde on a Saturday at euene
> Was pertliche for pruyde and for no poynt elles.
> Pere-trees and plum-trees were poffed to þe erthe
> In ensunple, segges, þat we sholde do þe bettere.
> Beches and brode okes were blowe to þe grounde
> And turned vpward here tayl in tokenynge of drede
> That dedly synne ar domesday shal fordon hem alle. (114–22)

Reason proves to the dreamer that pure sin causes pestilence. The storm Langland refers to is a famous storm that occurred on 15 January 1362 and was believed by many chroniclers to start the second outbreak of pestilence.[2] The Chronicle of Louth Park Abbey describes, "In A.D. 1361 there was a mortality of men, especially adolescents and boys, and as a result it was commonly called the pestilence of boys. In the same year, about the feast of St Maurus the abbot [15 January 1362] a strong gale blew from the north so violently for a day and night that it flattened trees, mills, houses, and a great many church towers" (Horrox 85–86). For Langland, both the pestilence and the storm are a representation of God's anger with man, and Langland believes it is his job to interpret the meaning of these events. However, a moral meaning of plague does not preclude a natural mechanism that brought plague about. And both moral and natural explanations about plague can be found not only in works of literature, but also in those of medicine and theology.

Langland's moral association between pestilence and sin may or may not come directly from medical authorities. Biblical sources about pestilence as a sign God's wrath are numerous: Exodus 9:14, Numbers 11:33, 2 Samuel 7:14, Psalms 89:23, 1 Samuel 4:8, and Isaiah 9:13. Nevertheless, Reason entertains some type of argument, for he "preuede" that pestilence comes from pride and "for no poynt elles." What other theories about plague does Reason disregard?

People of the Middle Ages believed in two possible causes for the plague: moral and natural. One the first chroniclers of the plague, Jacme d'Agramont wrote for the Crown of Aragon in Leria and published some of the earliest pamphlets on plague. These early texts provide the common medical attitudes and beliefs about bubonic plague "which was not to abandon Western Europe until the eighteenth century" (Arrizabalaga 238). In *Regiment de preservació de pestilència* (c.1348), Jacme d'Agramont provides a definition of moral pestilence: "Pestilence [morally understood] is a contranatural change (mundament) in the spirit and in the thoughts of people, resulting in enmities and rancours, wars and robberies, destruction of places and deaths far beyond the ordinary in certain regions" (qtd. in Arrizabalaga 245). Concerning this passage, Arrizabalaga states, "From Agramont's discussion of pestilences, the 'natural' and the 'moral' we may conclude ... [that] 'moral pestilence' was by no means just a metaphor. Agramont had no doubt about the existence of this kind of pestilence, so that his concept of *pestilència* was operative not only in the natural world, but also in a moral one" (245).

Natural pestilence, on the other hand, could be caused by earthquakes or contaminated water that released harmful gases into the air (Arrizabalaga 254–6). For example, Thomas Burton, a monk at Meaux Abbey located in Yorkshire, writes,

> At the beginning of 1349, during Lent on Friday before Passion Sunday [27 March], an earthquake was felt throughout England. Our monks at Meaux were at vespers and had come to the verse 'He hath put down the mighty' in the Magnificat, when they were thrown from their stalls by the earthquake and sent sprawling on the ground. The earthquake was quickly followed in this part of the country by the pestilence. (Horrox 68)

Henry Knighton, also a chronicler of the 1390s, concludes that all the deaths of pestilence "were brought about by the earthquake" (Horrox 77). Evidently, the earthquake theory of the origin of plague had considerable weight in England during Langland's time.

Reason may well be rejecting the medical community's earthquake theory regarding plague. By embracing the moral theory, Langland asserts that plague comes from a social, not cosmic level. Although Agramont and Langland see moral pestilence as a result of spiritual change, Langland believes that pestilence results from a turning toward pride, as we have seen in Passus XIII and XXII. Langland does not simply use a metaphor, but engages a social belief that sin could create plague.

Besides providing the "true" origin of pestilence, Langland also indicates the means of transmission. In Passus V, we notice that pestilence travels on "the south-weste wynde" (16). This information is not found in biblical sources but was believed by the medical community to have been a means of plague transmission. Medieval doctors believed that infection occurred when corrupt air or *miasma* from either natural sources or contagious people infiltrated the lungs which in turn affected the humors and the heart (Arrizabalaga 259–61; Gottfried, *Black Death*, 111). Gentile de Foligno, a fourteenth-century doctor who wrote an inventory of plague cures, explains the miasma theory: "The particular and manifest causes are the perceptible corruptions which are present at a place or carried in from distant places by means of winds, above all, by southerly ones" (qtd. in Arrizabalaga 255). Also, the Paris Medical Faculty in 1348 stated that the corrupted air is "spread abroad by frequent gusts of wind in the wild southerly gales"

(Horrox 161). Because doctors believed that pestilence was carried through the air, the first line of prevention was flight. However, if one was unable to flee, the individual needed to choose a place where ventilation could be controlled. As Arrizabalaga notes,

> The Paris masters advised moving one's house away from every place where putrefactions were copiously generated, such as 'marshy, muddy, and stinking places, stagnant waters and ditches,' ventilating it through windows open to northerly winds (as long as these did not pass through putrid and infected places), and protecting it from southerly ones because these were the usual carriers of pestilential air. (275)

John Jacobus, the royal and papal physician and Chancellor of Montpellier, also wrote a treatise on the Pestilence (c.1364) that was later translated into English. Concerning transmission, Jacobus writes:

> Also it is good for a patient to change his chamber every day and often to have the windows against the north and east and to spar the windows against the south. For the south wind has two causes of putrefaction. The first is it that makes a man, whether whole or sick, feeble in his body. The second cause is as it is written in Aphorisms, chapter 3, the south wind grieves the body and hurts the heart because it opens man's pores and enters into the heart. Wherefore it is good for a whole man in time of pestilence when the wind is in the south to stay within the house all day. (Horrox 176)

Since medical authorities believed pestilence was carried by the southerly winds and because there is no mention of southerly transmission in the Bible, one can infer that Langland was aware of common medical beliefs concerning plague transmission.

Langland demonstrates further medical knowledge regarding the natural forces that predict pestilence, such as astrological portents. Returning to Passus VIII, Langland predicts that plague will follow famine: "so sayth Saturne and sente vs to warne. / Throw flodes and thorw foule wederes fruyttes shollen fayle; / Pruyde and pestilences shal moche peple feche" (347–9). What is the relationship between Saturn and pestilence? Since pestilence devastated communities time and time again, doctors desired to predict future infections. Whether plague comes from natural or moral causes, astrological portents remained the same (Arrizabalaga 264). Like Isidore of Seville's investigation into the roots of words, doctors divided the word "pestilence" into three parts: "pes" equals "storm," "tempest" equals "time," and "leneia" equals "brightness" or "light." Therefore, the meaning of "pestilence" is the "time of the tempest caused by the light of the stars" (Arrizabalaga 244). Doctors believed that light created by certain celestial alignments corrupted the air. Consequently, medical knowledge regarding astrology and astronomy increased in order to predict future pestilences.

Doctors believed that the alignment of Jupiter, a warm and moist planet, and Mars, a hot and dry planet, were the root cause of pestilence. When this alignment occurred, Mars ignited the excessive moisture from Jupiter and these rays rained down on the earth thus affecting the miasma (Campbell 40). However, Saturn also figured into this portent, as he does in *Piers Plowman*. As Gottfried attests, "No one was quite sure what Saturn had or did, but most experts felt that its combination with anything was bad" (*Black Death*, 111).

Chaucer, Langland's contemporary, may help structure Saturn's role in relation to pestilence. In the *Knight's Tale*, Saturn states to his daughter Venus, "My lookyng is the fader of pestilence" (I. 2469). Since Chaucer was the first person to translate an astrological work into the vernacular, namely *A Treatise on the Astrolabe* (c.1391), we can assume that he was knowledgeable of contemporary astrological learning. Therefore, on the authority of Chaucer, we learn that Saturn foretold the coming of pestilence. However, Langland's use of this information does not mean that he is questioning the moral nature of plague by referring to natural causes. Astrological signs are often used by medical doctors to forecast plague, regardless of whether it is moral or natural plague (Arrizabalaga 252). In fact the report by the Paris Medical Faculty after the outbreak of the first plague states, "The mortality of races and the depopulation of kingdoms occur at the conjunction of Saturn and Jupiter" (Horrox 159). Similarly, in *On the Judgment of Sol at the Feasts of Saturn*, Simone de Covino writes, "Saturn puts forward reasons for the destruction of the human race and Jupiter puts forward a defence to them" (Horrox 165). Geoffrey de Meaux also offers an astrological reason for the pestilence: "I do not wish to imply that the mortality comes only from Saturn and Jupiter but rather through Mars, which was mixed with them at the time of the eclipse" (Horrox 171). While Langland uses natural predictions of plague, he never wavers from his belief that pestilence is God's wrath for human sins.

Edward III argued that plague had a moral cause in a letter to the bishops in 1349: "For we hope that if, by God's grace, the people drive out this spiritual wickedness from their hearts, the malignancy of the air and of the other elements will also depart" (Horrox 118). According to both Edward and Langland, the cure is within the hands of the people who simply need to repent their sins. When that occurs, God will remove the natural causes that brought about plague. Moreover, the Paris Medical Faculty ends their treatise on pestilence by saying: "We must not overlook the fact that any pestilence proceeds from the divine will, and our advice can therefore only be to return humbly to God" (Horrox 163). Similarly, Jacobus states, "A man ought to forsake evil things and do good deeds and meekly confess his sins, for it is the highest remedy in time of pestilence: penance and confession to be preferred to all other medicine" (Horrox 176). Evidently, medicine, theology, and literature were all attempting to find a unified reason for this disease's visitation. A natural cause, therefore, does not preclude a divine reason.

While Langland identifies the causes of plague, the means of transmission, and the means of forecasting future occurrences, he also provides ways to avoid sickness through behavioral changes, particularly dietary modifications. In Passus VIII, Langland advocates dietary moderation as a way to prevent illness. After Hunger corrects Wastor's followers, Piers asks Hunger, "Yf ȝe can or knowe eny kyne thynges of fisyk, / For somme of my seruauntes and mysulf bothe / Of al a woke worche nat, so oure wombe greueth vs" (VIII. 227–9). Hunger replies by telling Piers:

> Y wot wel, ... what sekenesse ȝow ayleth.
> ȝe han manged ouer-moche—þat maketh ȝow to be syke.
> Ac ete nat, y hote, ar hunger the take
> And sende the of his sauce to sauery with thy lyppes.
> And kepe som til soper tyme and site nat to longe
> At noon ne at no tyme, and nameliche at þe sopere
> Lat nat sire Sorfeet sittien at thy borde,
> And loke þou drynke no day ar thow dyne sumwhat. (VIII. 271–78)

To be healthy, Piers and the fair field of folk must practice dietary moderation. They must not eat or drink too much and should not sit at the table too long. This dietary information echoes Holy Church's belief that "mesure is medecyne" (I. 33). By practicing both a dietary and work regimen, Hunger states that the fair field of folk will be free of disease. Significantly, Hunger describes a dietary regimen similar to that prescribed by doctors as a precaution against plague.

Doctors also advocated dietary and work modifications so that infected air would not dramatically change the humeral balance. Relying on Galen, Gentile de Foligno suggests, "[I]f someone works moderately and leads a decorous life, he will be able to remain untouched [by the pestilence]" (qtd. in Arrizabalaga 273). However, Gentile states that those at greatest risk are "those full of superfluities and those of inactive men, copious eaters and drinkers" (qtd. in Arrizabalaga 279). Plague doctors, both in England and on the Continent, advocated moderation, specifically in diet. They often suggested that a person should leave the table hungry and should avoid rich foods (Arrizabalaga 279). Likewise, John of Burgundy's 1365 treatise on plague states: "First, you should avoid over-indulgences in food and drink ... and should consume easily-digested food and spiced wine diluted with water" (Horrox 186). These preventative measures are markedly similar to Holy Church's statement that measure is medicine and Hunger's suggestion of dietary and labor regimen. Both Langland and doctors focus on the need for individuals to recognize and change their behaviors in order to avoid plague.

However, Langland implies that if the individual will not control his or her own behavior, a social superior must take over. The relationship Langland suggests between medicine and rural practice is not uncommon. When Piers asks Hunger to provide some medical information so that Piers can keep his fair field of folk healthy, Piers acts much like a landlord of the fair field of folk. Recent scholarship has shown that medicine was often included within rural estate handbooks because of the unavailability of university-trained physicians. Studying Peter of Cresent's *Twelve Books on Rural Practices* (ca. 1230), William C. Crossgrove attests, "Peter wants to suggest that if academic physicians are not available, the next best thing is for the educated estate manager to provide treatment using the knowledge that has been accumulated by academic medicine" (99). While Langland employs academic medical beliefs, he does not imply that landlords are better than doctors are. Instead, Langland's medicine centers on the moral failure of the individual and the authoritative nature of the landlord. For Langland, people become sick because they lack moderation, specifically by eating too much and not doing enough work enough. Therefore, the landlord needs to structure the worker's life. The benefits of moderation will, as Hunger states, improve both the individual and the community:

> And yf thow dyete the thus y dar legge myn eres
> That Fysik shal his forred hodes for his fode sulle
> And his cloke of Callabre for his comune legge
> And be fayn, be my fayth, his fysik to leete
> And lerne to labor with lond lest lyflode hem fayle. (VIII.290–4)

For Hunger, a sinful life leads to sickness. Without sin, there would be no sickness and doctors would need to find new means of employment. While Langland's syllogism is hopelessly utopian, it does identify the importance he places on changing one's behavior.

Langland not only identifies the causes of plague but also identifies how certain social groups fail to alter their morally deficient behavior. David Aers explains, "For Langland the search for God is certainly bound up with the search for a just community and a reformed Church, a search constantly engaging with specific contemporary problems and conflicts" (*Culture* 184). Since the Black Death did not discriminate among social classes or among the pious and non-pious, one wonders how Langland interprets the victimization of pious individuals. In Passus III, Langland states that good must also be punished with the bad, but that the innocent will be rewarded in heaven:

> That so bigileth hem of here goed, þat god on hem sende
> Feuer or fouler euel other fuyr on here houses,
> Morreyne or other meschaunces; and mony tymes hit falleth
> That innocence is herde in heuene amonge seyntes
> That louten for hem to oure lorde and to oure lady bothe. (III. 98–102)

In other words, the innocent are often lost with the guilty. God will grant the innocent heavenly reward, while the guilty must endure punishment in hell.

To avoid punishment in hell, God "graunte gylours on erthe grace to amende" (III. 103).

As we have seen, Langland believed that sin created pestilence. However, the bubonic plague caused social changes by placing more money in fewer hands and by creating job opportunities. The amends Langland offers the society are a rejection of monetary wealth caused by labor changes and bequests.[3] As Aers notes, "These [labor] changes offered opportunities for landless labourers, craftsmen, and many peasants, opportunities to improve the extremely vulnerable existence on the margins of survival led by their ancestors in the previous 150 years" (*Community*, 26). Langland's ideas about the plague are caught in a paradox. The increase in wealth led to an increase in worldly goods and an increase in sin. Therefore, pestilence may be seen as an effective individual deterrent, since those who die can never sin again. But it is an ineffective social deterrent, since it increases monetary sins. Langland confirms the paradoxical nature of pestilence in Passus XI:

> That folk is nat ferme in þe faith ne fre of here godes
> Ne sory for here synnes; so ys pruyde enhanced
> In religion and in al þe reume amonges rich and pore
> That preyeres haen no power this pestilences to lette.
> For gode is deef nowadays and deyneth vs nat to here
> And gode men for oure gultes he al togrynt to deth.
> And ȝut this wreches of this world, is noen ywar by oþer,
> Ne for drede of eny deth withdraweth hym fro pruyde
> Ne parteth with þe pore, as puyr charite wolde,
> Bote in gaynesse and in glotonye forglotten here godes
> And breketh nat here bred to þe pore. (57–66)

Even though people know that sin causes pestilence, few modified their behavior: "ne for drede of eny deth withdraweth fro pruyde." Aers states, "For Langland the profit economy he saw pervading social relations and spiritual relations was the source and embodiment of much he detested and feared in his own search for a just and stable community responsive to the call of Christ" ("Class" 69). What Langland detests and fears is a society that knows the causes of pestilence and still fails to modify its sinful nature. Therefore, Langland focuses on specific social groups, such as doctors, clergy, and beggars, all of whom received monetary rewards created by the Black Death.

While Langland uses university medicine to defend his theory of the plague, he attacks the medical community for its ineffectiveness and greed. Their potions are said to kill; Hunger states, "There ar many luther leches ac lele leches fewe; / That don men deye thorw here drynkes ar destyne hit wolde" (VIII. 295–96). Much of the resentment toward doctors may be attributed to the medical community's inability to control pestilence. While the bubonic plague did not invalidate the entire force of medicine, it did raise questions regarding classical medical theory, education, and practice (Siraisi, *Medieval*, 42–43). One reason why medicine may not have been damaged by the plague is that mortality rates of recurrent plagues were less and less. From the perspective of the layperson, this would imply that the medical community's handling of this disease was improving.

However, during the plague years, the lay population often condemned doctors for getting rich off of an incurable disease. As Conscience states, "Harlotes and hoores and also fals leches / They asken here huyre ar thei haue deserued" (III. 300–01). Interestingly, Langland compares the monetary value of sex to that of medicine. The aspect that unifies this comparison is the perversion of love. Whores and harlots pervert sex because they charge for their love. Similarly, false doctors charge money for an illness that could be cured by love: "For Treuthe telleth þat loue ys triacle to abate synne / And the most souerayne salue for soule and for body" (I. 147–48). Since Langland believes that illness is caused by sin and sin is alleviated through an herbal (triacle) called love, doctors, like harlots, pervert a natural act by charging for the cure. This perversion can only be changed if doctors forego worldly gains or if people change their sinfulness and thereby no longer become sick.

The criticism of doctors for charging more than they should does have some social validity. Like Langland, Chaucer makes a reference to plague doctors and greed. The narrator of *The Canterbury Tales* characterizes the Physician thus: "And yet he was but esy of dispence; / He kepte that he wan in pestilence. / For gold in phisik is a cordial, / Therefore, he loved gold in special" (I. 441–44). Doctors did indeed make money off of pestilence. Often their prevention and cures depended on the social class of the infected individuals. Arrizabalaga concludes,

> Both Gentile de Foligno and the Paris masters in their curative regimes offered a range of the therapeutic preparations directed to different social groups. The most significant example of this may be the potion that Gentile suggested to those who were 'rich and wealthy enough': it consisted of barley water which had to be boiled with gold straw (*virga auri*) before serving as the basis for preparing various dishes (*fercula*). (285)

Besides expensive cures, plague doctors offered preventative steps that could be taken to fumigate corrupt air. Often these measures centered on Galen's belief that aromatic fumes kept people healthy. The choice of plants and woods to be burned also related to the person's social class. For the poor, Gentile suggested very cheap herbs such as marjoram, savory, and mint. On the other hand, the Paris Masters recommended very expensive substances, wood of aloes, amber, and musk, for "the rich and powerful" (Arrizabalaga 275). While neither cures nor preventative measures helped to alleviate or prevent infection, they do demonstrate that doctors took advantage of the patient's social standing. Since these remedies did not work, it is not surprising to find lay people such as Langland and Chaucer expressing hostility toward the monetary rewards of plague doctors. But for Langland, this is another representation of the sinful nature of his society that needs to be modified.

Doctors are not the only people Langland attacks for pursuing monetary rewards after the Black Death; he also attacks the clergy for choosing money over service. Langland's attack on the clergy focuses on two different groups: priests that take advantage of civic jobs and priests who are unqualified to hold the position. In the *Prologue*, Langland condemns priests who take civic jobs because parish jobs are monetarily unrewarding:

> Persones and parsches prestis pleyned to þe bischop
> That here parasches were pore sithe þe pestelence tyme,
> To haue a licence and a leue in Londoun to dwelle
> And synge þer for symonye while seluer is so swete.
> Bishopes and bachelers, bothe maystres and doctours,
> That han cure vnder Crist and crownyng in tokene
> And ben charged with holy chirche charite to tylie,
> That is lele loue and lyfe among lered and lewed,
> Leyen in Londoun in lenton and elles.
> Summe seruen þe kyng and his siluer tellen,
> In þe cheker and in þe chancerye chalengen his dettes
> Of wardus and of wardemotis, wayues and strayues;
> And summe aren as seneschalles and seruen oþer lordes
> And ben in stede of stewardus and sitten and demen. (85–95)[4]

By taking civic jobs, parish priests worshiped worldly over heavenly goods and, therefore, continued to sin. Furthermore, they left their parishes untended thereby increasing the possibility of sin. The Black Death did indeed leave many parishes unattended, since pestilence struck the ecclesiastical orders harder than other social orders. While most other social orders suffered about thirty-percent mortality, the ecclesiastical community suffered forty- to fifty-percent. As Gottfried attests,

> Mortality among the clergy in England seems to have been even higher than that among the lay population. In Somerset, the diocese just south of Bath and Wells, admission to new benefices rose over 500% from November 1348 to January 1349. In Oxford, 43% of the beneficed clergy died. In Bicester, about 13 miles northeast of Oxford, 40% of the beneficed clergy perished, while in Wycombe, in Buckinghamshire, it was an astonishing 66%. (*Black Death*, 62)

Pestilence struck the clerical orders the hardest because of the nature of their jobs. The necessity for the parish priest to hear confessions, to administer last rites to plague victims, and to live in poorer conditions in comparison to higher clergy would have increased the chance of flea contact (Courtenay 703). Furthermore, if clergy were being decimated by the disease and medieval people believed that the disease was God's wrath, then by logical indirection, the priests are sinful, too. Hays writes, "And even if a clergyman remained devoted to his parish in its travail, his powerlessness was manifest; the extent to which members of the clergy commanded respect because of their 'superhuman' qualities was weakened by their inability to stem the disease, and by their vulnerability to it" (50).

The reduction in the population of priests opened avenues of civic employment such as chantries that provided many priests with handsome incomes and political civic rewards. "Chantries provided jobs," writes Courtenay, "and many of these went to priests with university backgrounds" (713). University priests who took civic jobs further reduced the number of available priests already decimated by the Black Death. In response to the high mortality rate and the need for trained priests, admission rates to dioceses dramatically increased. Unfortunately, the mass production of priests is not as easy as the replacement of common laborers. As Courtenay states, "We have many references after 1348 to vacancies and the appointment of less qualified candidates" (707). The lack of parish priests became so great that it forced the Bishop of Bath and Wells to write in 1349:

> The contagious pestilence of the present day, which is spreading far and wide, has left many parish churches without parson or priest to care for the parishioners. Since no priests can be found who are willing, whether out of zeal or devotion to exchange for a stipend, to take pastoral care of these aforesaid places, not to visit the sick and administer to them the sacraments of the church, we understand that many people are dying without the sacrament of penance. [Therefore] ... persuade all men, in particular, those who are now sick or should feel sick in the future, that, if they are on the point of death and cannot secure the services of a priest, then they should make confession to each other ... or if no man is present, then even to a woman. (qtd. in Gottfried, *Black Death*, 62)

As continued occurrences of the plague took more lives, other methods of handling last rites became common. For example, Thomas Walsington, a monk, chronicled the fourth and fifth pestilences between 1376 and 1392. He writes, "Meanwhile as the plague raged in England, Pope Clement granted—because of the epidemic—full remission of penance to all those throughout the kingdom who died truly contrite and after making confession" (Horrox 66). The death of beneficed clergy, the movement of parish priests to civic jobs, the mass production of new clergy, and the insistence that lay people could perform confession and last rites created questions about the authority and power of the Church.

Langland recognized that the mass production of priests had placed many unlearned men in positions of power and that these priests were often as sinful as the communities they are suppose to save. While there are many references in *Piers Plowman* to unlearned priests, two should suffice: the characterization of Sloth as a "prest and persoun passynge thritty wyntur" and not knowing the "*pater-noster*" (VII. 10–30) and the mention that "lewede" priests lead men to sin (XIV. 123–24). But the social problems caused by unlearned priests goes deeper than just leading men to sin. Like the priests that move to chantries in the city, the parish priests also commit worldly sins by desiring "suluer" (XVI. 276) and misappropriating funds: "Y dar nat carpe of clerkes now þat Cristes tresor kepe / That pore peple by puyre riht her part myhte aske" (XVII. 68–69). These priests sin because they desire worldly over heavenly rewards. As Langland sees it, people can no longer rely on the clerical order to provide a proper moral structure. However, if the ecclesiastical order would right itself, if it would recognize and change its sinful behaviors, society would improve: "ȝf prestes doen here deuer wel we shal do þe bettere" (XVII.122). Langland identifies behaviors of priests that put the society at risk of further punishments by God and calls for the ecclesiastical orders to change those behaviors.

Besides doctors and priests, Langland also blames beggars for preferring sin to moderation. As plague reduced the population, many middle-class survivors became wealthy. This increased charitable giving. Gottfried notes, "In England, about a quarter of all testators' estates, land, and movables, went to good works ... 70 new [hospital] foundations were laid between 1350 and 1390" (*Black Death* 85). Unfortunately, the increase in charity created a situation in which many healthy individuals could make more money begging than working. For Langland, the increase of beggars is an increase in sin because they are gluttons: "Bidders and beggers fast aboute ȝede / Til here bagge and here bely was bretful ycrammed, / Fayteden for here fode and foughten at þe ale" (*Prol.* 42–45).[5] Furthermore, beggars increase sin because they are slothful and do not work. Langland narrates the civic authority's response to healthy beggars. In Passus VIII, Piers confronts the workers that feign illness:

> ȝe been wastours, y woet wel, and waste and deuouren
> What lele land-tilynge men leely byswynken.
> Ac Treuthe shal teche ȝow his teme to dryue
> Or ȝe shal ete barly breed and of þe broke drynke,
> But yf he be blynde or broke-legged or bolted with yren—
> Suche poore,' quod Peres, 'shal parte with my godes,
> Bothe of my corn and of my cloth to kepe hem fram defaute. (135–45)

Piers does not forbid physically injured people from begging but instead attacks those wasters that feign injury so as not to work. But the beggar's spokesperson, Wastor, takes no heed of Piers's indictment and tells Piers to "go pisse with his plogh" (151). Piers then takes legal action by calling for the knight, who warns Wastor to work "or y shal bette the by the lawe and brynge þe in stokkes" (163).[6] Wastor ignores the law and his followers are not brought to work until Hunger attacks.

Langland describes the social events caused by the bubonic plague. The increase in charity and the increase in beggars forced the legal establishment to enact laws against people "preferring to be in idleness rather than by labor to get their living" (Krochalis 78). The end of the King's Proclamation Concerning Laborers (1351) sums up the problems caused by increased charity and prohibits giving to able bodied beggars:

> And because that many strong beggars, as long as they may live begging, do refuse to labor, giving themselves to idleness and vice, and sometimes to theft and other abominations; none upon the said pain of imprisonment, shall, under the color of pity or alms, give anything to such, which may labor, or presume to favor them in idleness, so that thereby they may be compelled to labor for their necessary living. (qtd. in Krochalis 79)

To remain in idleness when healthy is to sin. Therefore, the civic authority sought through poll taxes to distinguish between the "true" beggar and the "false," between the healthy and the lame (Dyer 252). But as Langland's poem makes evident, human law was ineffective at modifying or controlling behaviors. These behaviors only change when threatened by natural law, the law of survival. Hunger forces the people to work and to renounce sin. Pestilence, Langland believes, should have the same effect.

Women were also not immune to Langland's attack; he admonishes them for not replenishing the supply of humans. In 1350, one of the earliest chroniclers of the plague writes, "Most of the women who survived remained barren for many years. If any did conceive they generally died, along with the baby, in giving birth" (Horrox 64). Recurrent pandemics continued to keep the population low. In fact, not until the sixteenth century would the population exceed its 1350 high (Gottfried, *Black Death*, xvi). Langland clearly recognized the need to repopulate. But before repopulating could occur, people had to overcome their sinful nature. As Langland sees it, too many married people bicker and fight, and the couples marry for reasons other than love:

> In ielosye, ioyles, and iangelynge abedde,
> Many a payre sethe this pestelences han plyhte treuthe to louye,
> Ac they lyen lely, here neyther lyketh other.
> The fruyt þat they brynge forth aren many foule wordes;
> Haen þei no childerne bute cheste and choppes hem bitwene.
> Thogh they do hem to Donemowe, bote þe deuel hem helpe,
> To folwe for þe flicche, fecheth they hit neuere;
> Bote they bothe be forswore þat bacon þei tyne. (X. 269–75)

Langland's call for repopulating is once again caught in a social and psychological paradox. Some marriages no longer produced children, but money. Since some people would marry for money and not love, they continued to breed sin and "destroy the nuclear family, already unquestionably traditional amongst the great majority of the population" (Aers, *Community* 52). For Langland, the search for monetary reward in marriage created sin and few offspring. Chaucer demonstrates a similar belief in his characterization of the Wife of Bath, who has been married five times and appears to be childless.

Langland was not alone in his criticism of women and their desire for money. John of Reading, a chronicler of the 1361 pestilence writes, "The greatest cause of grief was provided by the behaviour of women. Widows, forgetting the love they had borne towards their husbands, rushed into the arms of foreigners or, in many cases, of kinsmen, and shamelessly gave birth to bastards conceived in adultery" (Horrox 87). Interestingly, Langland's opinion about fruitful marriages seems to have some social validity. Peasant families of the late fourteenth century were considerably smaller than those of pre-plague years (Dyer 146). The aristocracy also had difficulty reproducing, as Gottfried notes, "In England, 75% of all noble families failed to produce a male heir through two generations. This meant continual flux among the aristocracy as old families died out and new ones replaced them" (*Black Death* 96).[7] For Langland, only by correcting sins of society, especially a desire for worldly wealth, would human beings abate God's wrath and recover from the plague's decimation.

Unlike Boccaccio's demonstration of frivolity, sexual excess, and hedonism, Langland's satire provides a somber interpretation of pestilence. Geoffrey Shepard concludes about Langland's work: "There must be recognition of what has gone wrong, then society must commit itself wholeheartedly to a purer intention and devise and pursue just and effective policies" (169). In one sense, *Piers Plowman* can be read as a prescription for curing plague. Aers states, "The vision [Langland offers] is a stirring affirmation of human solidarity, one whose survival now seems bound up with the very survival of the earth and its people" (*Community* 67). Langland concludes that pestilence is a sign from God that should correct man's sins.

GEOFFREY CHAUCER'S *THE PARDONER'S TALE*

While Langland isolates the sin of pride as the cause of the plague, other authors focus on other sins. While it would appear that Chaucer mentions the plague only in passing, his choice of setting is important. Peter Beidler states, "Of all the early tellers of the famous story of evil men whose greed leads them to their death after finding a pile of gold, Chaucer alone places his version in plague times" (257). The Pardoner demonstrates the frailty of life during time of plague when he has one of the rioters come out of a tavern to wonder about the corpse's name in the passing funeral (661–9). The rioter sends a servant to find out the name of the corpse, and the servant replies,

> ... it nedeth never-a-deel;
> It was told er ye cam heer two houres.
> He was, pardee, an old felawe of youres,
> And sodeynly he was yslayn to-night
> Fordronke, as he sat on his bench upright.
> Ther cam a privee theef men clepeth Deeth,
> That in this contree all the peple sleeth,
> And with his spere he smoot his herte atwo,
> And wente his wey withouten wordes mo.
> He hath a thousand slayn this pestilence. (670–9)

Concerning this passage, Beidler points out that the plague is not a one-time occurrence, but that the boy is referring to "this pestilence" which "suggests there had been earlier visitations of pestilence in that area" (258). Furthermore, in relation to health regimens in the face of plague, the *Tale*'s exemplum suggests that those who drink copiously are more at risk of plague. A modification of drinking and eating habits is also the first preventative action mentioned by the medical doctor John of Burgundy in 1365. Burgundy writes: "First, you should avoid over-indulgences in food and drink" (Horrox 186). By connecting pestilence to drinking, Chaucer is also providing his readers with preventative methods and explaining what type of person the plague is seeking. In other words, the man who died of plague brought it on himself because he failed to modify his drinking. Beidler writes, "Such actions and attitudes were surely perceived by sensible observers as both sinful and suicidal, but all accounts suggest that in showing his rioters carousing in a tavern, Chaucer was merely being a realist, for such behavior was apparently common" (259). More importantly, this behavior allows the readers to separate themselves from those infected because they may not be part of the social group that this disease is targeting.[8] But Chaucer is not content merely to connect copious drinkers to the scourge of pestilence. Instead, he expands the list of potential sinners to include all listening to the Pardoner's words. What is different between Chaucer and Langland is that Chaucer does not allow for innocence. All of the parties in *The Pardoner's Tale* are guilty of sin, and so too is the entire audience.

If one believes that plague is sent by God to correct man's sin, part of man's job is to interpret which sin is God trying to correct. At least one chronicler states that the pestilence was a punishment for false oaths, which also seems to be the connection between the *Pardoner's Tale* and its setting. Sloane MS 965 is a collection of medical and astrological texts. In the manuscript, the medical treatise by John of Burgundy (1365) on pestilence is followed by an anonymous tract on the sins that have brought about pestilence. After the author cites numerous biblical examples of retribution by God, such as the stories of Lucifer, Moses and Aaron, Noah, and Sodom and Gomorrah, he connects the biblical stories to the bubonic plague. The author writes:

> When a powerful pestilence reigned in the land of David because it had not obeyed the commands of God, to which King Solomon referred: 'He that sweareth much shall be filled with iniquity: and a scourge shall not depart from his house' [Ecclesiasticus 23.12]. And it therefore follows from these examples that pestilence arises from a multitude of sins, but most especially from swearing worthless, deceitful and meaningless oaths. (Horrox 193)

The connection between false oaths and disease must have been an important line of reasoning throughout the Middle Ages, because both leprosy and plague were connected to false oaths and blasphemy.

Chaucer's tale is an exemplum, which raises the question, what example is it giving to the readers, especially in relation to plague? I believe Chaucer, like Langland, is making a social statement that identifies sin as the cause of the pestilence. The sin Chaucer seems to identify as the cause of plague is false oaths, both oaths made from man to man and from man to God. Other literary critics have proposed that the Pardoner is identifying the tavern sins or Pride as the most recognizable sin in the tale. Helen Cooper writes, "The homiletic material at the start of the tale draws on a variety of sources. The sins of gluttony and drunkenness, gambling ('hazardrye'), and blasphemy, collectively known as the 'tavern sins,' were favourite subjects of preachers and moralists" (265). While the tavern sins do seem to be logical choices, it would also seems that blaming only one group, in this case the drinkers, would be too specific and would not prompt sufficient internal reflection for Chaucer's readers.

The rioters think that they "wol sleen this false traytour Deeth" (699), an act equivalent to Christ's resurrection. One could read this exemplum as criticizing people's Pride in relation to pestilence. Concerning the rioters, Derek Pearsall writes:

> The rioters' decision to go out in search of Death in order to slay him is made in a spirit of drunken bravado: it is not the act of public-spirited vigilantes but, in the context of Christian understanding that presses imperatively for recognition in the tale, a sign of moral deadness, as well as a grotesque parody of Christ's struggle to overcome Death, which brought about of course not the elimination of physical death but the release of man from certainty of eternal damnation. (*Canterbury* 101)

The exemplum does reflect a moral deadness on the part of the rioters. But the moral deadness needs to be general in order to allow the audience to reflect on the merits of the tale as well as to see their reflection in actions of the rioters. Consequently, I doubt that the exemplum examines the role of pride because it is too specific for few readers have literally or metaphorically attempted to kill death.

The sin that I think Chaucer is identifying is partly connected to the tavern sins, but is much more common to a general audience: the sin of swearing false oaths. False oaths could fall under blasphemy in Cooper's argument; however, I believe that Chaucer is pointing to a more social reading of false oaths. The Pardoner defines blasphemy when he says:

> But ydel sweryng is a cursednesse.
> Bihoold and se that in the first table
> Of heighe Goddes heestes honourable,
> Hou that the second heeste of hym is this:
> 'Take nat my name in ydel or amys'
> Lo, rather he forbedeth swich sweryng
> Than homycide or many a cursed thyng. (638–44)

The rioters do much swearing and cursing that could be seen as blasphemous; however, there is an interesting structure in *The Pardoner's Tale* that seems to suggest that pacts made between men are to be considered as important as those made between man and God.

After the rioters decide to seek out Death and kill him, and once again commit blasphemy by saying, "By Goddes dignitee" (701), the narrator explains the following events:

> Togidres han thise thre hir trouthes plight
> To lyve and dyen ech of hem for oother,
> As thoguh he were his owene ybore brother.
> And up they stirte, al droken in this rage,
> And forth they goon towardes that village
> Of which the taverner hadde spoke biforn.
> And many risly ooth thanne han they sworn,
> And Cristes blessed body they torente—
> Death shal be deed, if that they may hym hente (702–10).

Cursing to God contextualizes the pledge the rioters make. Cooper argues, "The threat [to kill Death] is also a powerful example of a pervasive motif of the tale—the reduction of the spiritual to the physical, such as has been shown already by the Pardoner in his Prologue. The destruction of Death is taken as a material quest" (269). However, the pact made between the rioters is elevated from the physical to the spiritual, as it is that pact which is broken and causes their death. What rends God's heart is the same that rends man's heart—falseness. The rioters make two oaths, one to God and one to Christ, before making their pact with each other. Their pact is to seek out and kill Death and to protect each other as sworn brothers. The realm of sworn brothers is elevated from the physical to the spiritual by swearing the pact with oaths to God.

The rioters do not protect each other as brothers, nor do they succeed in their quest to find Death and kill him. Instead, they are distracted by "floryns fyne of gold yconyned rounde / Wel ny an eighte busshels, as hem thoughte"

(770–1). The narrator underscores the effect of this distraction, "No lenger thann after Deeth they sought" (772). Thus the first oath to find Death has been broken. The second oath to protect each other as brothers is broken when the two rioters send the third to get food and drink. While the rioter in search of sustenance is gone, the other two plot to kill him upon his return (808–836). Interestingly, one rioter opens his suggestion of murder by saying, "Thow knowest wel thou art my sworen brother" (808), and ends the passage, "Hadde I nat doon a freendes torn to thee?" (815). This rioter affirms his oath of fidelity, an oath taken by all three rioters at the beginning of the tale. It would now appear that the oath to protect all three as sworn brothers has been broken by another oath between two rioters wanting to protect each other.

The rioter that has gone for food decides to poison the wine so that he can have all the money. In this, he breaks his oath to the others. He goes to an apothecary and explains that "... ther was a polcat in his hawe / That, as he seyde, his capouns hadde yslawe" (855–6). According to the *Physiologus*, the polecat, more commonly known as the weasel, gives birth through the ears, and the anonymous author states that this represents that "wicked things are engendered through the ears" (XXXV, Curley trans.). The relationship between the weasel and human beings is that human beings are deaf to the words of others, especially God. The narrator of the *Physiologus* states, "There are those even now eating the spiritual bread in church. When they have been dismissed, however, they will cast the Word out of their hearing" (XXXV, Curley trans.). The connection between the weasel and the rioters is that neither hear the words that are spoken, either to God in the blasphemous oaths they utter or to man in the social contracts they make. The rioters swear brotherhood, but do not remember what that means. Making false oaths, at least according to the Pardoner, appears to bring about death for the rioters.

In *Social Chaucer*, Paul Strohm states, "[Chaucer's] most trenchant examinations of the practice link false swearing with the falsification of human ties, as in the *Pardoner's Tale*. There Chaucer produces a travesty both of brotherhood and of the oaths that support it" (97). Strohm continues by explaining that the holding of hands when making their oaths "while something short of an *immixio manum*, is nevertheless a gesture toward solemnization" (97). The solemnization of the oaths and the men's failure is more than the result of a changing economic structure in which social hierarchies are shifting from a vertical feudal hierarchy to horizontal communal relationship (Strohm x). It can also be seen in relation to the plague that sits behind the Pardoner's setting of his tale about false oaths.

The importance of sworn brotherhood is not uncommon to Chaucer's work. As Strohm has shown, not only does the *Pardoner's Tale* contemplate brotherhood, so do the *Friar's* and *Summoner's Tales*, "but within a more particularized historical frame" (97). Strohm concludes, "Embedded in each are feudal concepts and norms, invoked not with nostalgic but with ironic intent, to underscore their supplantation by more self-interested alliances"

(97–8). At least for the *Pardoner's Tale*, sworn brotherhood may also be a temporary belief about the cause of plague that Chaucer chooses to dramatize. Since the *Pardoner's Tale* is an exemplum, Chaucer does not have the Pardoner name the characters of the tale because, like Langland's Plowman, the rioters are meant to reflect all of Chaucer's readers. The readers are meant to contemplate their own broken oaths and how those acts have continued the pestilence and God's anger.

THE YORK CYCLE: *MOSES AND PHARAOH*

In the York Corpus Christi play, the dramatist anachronistically mentions bubonic plague during the tale of the slaughter of the innocents. Like the mention of bubonic plague in Chaucer's *The Pardoner's Tale*, the mention of plague in the York cycle also relates to the sin of false oaths. More importantly, the mention of plague by the York dramatist seems to recall an outbreak of plague that struck only children. Richard Beadle begins his discussion of the York cycle by examining *Moses and Pharaoh*:

> In chapter 12 of the book of Exodus, God's final vengeance upon the Egyptians for the enslavement of the children of Israel is the death of the firstborn. Called upon to mention the incident in the play of *Moses and Pharaoh*, a writer in medieval York chose to substitute 'grete pestelence' for the biblical episode, a striking alteration to the canonical source, for in later medieval England 'the grete pestelence' had come to be the customary way of referring to the Black Death of 1348–9. (85)

Beadle believes that when the audience viewed this play, they may have used this reference as a type of remembrance for those who died of plague (85). Beadle suggests that plague was a one-time event, and that by the time 1376, a possible date for the earliest performance of the York cycle, the plague was only a distant memory to the medieval audience.[9] While the dates for the performance of this play remain uncertain, the reoccurrence of plague makes this play seem more timely to the audience than Beadle may realize.

According to the *Anonimalle Chronicles*, the fourth pestilence that struck England between 1374–9 affected numerous cites in both the north and south of England. One of the towns singled out for the devastation to its community was York. The chronicle reads: "In 1378 the fourth pestilence arrived in York and was particularly fatal to children. It began there before Michaelmas [29 September] and lasted for over a year" (Horrox 88). Since York was struck with a plague around the time of the writing of the play, and since the plague seems to have affected children more than adults, it would seem logical that the York *Moses and Pharaoh* play include pestilence, especially since the biblical story is about a plague that takes children. Furthermore, the play reinforces common beliefs about the role of false oaths in relation to the presence of plague.

Moses and Pharaoh opens by identifying a problem with progeny. The Second Counselor tells Pharaoh:

> The Jews that won here in Goshen
> And are named the children of Israel
> They multiply so fast
> That soothly we suppose
> They are like, and they last,
> Your lordship for to lose. (31–6)

The Counselor demonstrates a fear of culture and a change in the power of the ruling class. Unlike Pharaoh's culture, the Jews, members of the lower class, somehow produce children faster than the upper class. Consequently, the Jews would eventually outnumber the Egyptians and take over the land. This is a common social fear about marginalized groups: their breeding practices are more productive than the group in power. Pharaoh underscores the interest in their breeding practices when he responds: "What devil ever may it mean / That they so fast increase?" (47–8). Pharaoh decides that he can slow down the population increase of the Jews by making the

> . . . midwives to spill them
> When our Hebrews are born,
> All that are man-kind, to kill them;
> So shall they soon be lorn. (69–72)

In other words, this plague that Pharaoh sets up is a man-made plague, one that is designed to keep the Jewish population in check.

While Pharaoh plans a plague, God expresses to Moses His wishes for the people of Israel. God explains that He wants Moses to tell Pharaoh to "let my people pass / That they to wilderness may wend" (125–26). Moses reminds God that the Pharaoh "will not to me trast / For all the oaths that I may swear" (139–40). The mention of swearing oaths demonstrates the untrustworthiness among men. Moses fears that Pharaoh and his people will not heed the word of God as explained through Moses' mouth. God encourages Moses by saying, "And if thou might not move ne mum / I shall thee save from sin and shame" (175–76). God will protect Moses by making sure that neither Moses' actions nor words bring shame or sin. In other words, God molds human actions in order to do divine bidding.

While Pharaoh plans destruction, God speaks to Moses about the prosperity of the people of Israel. Because Pharaoh does not heed Moses' warnings from God, God punishes the Egyptians with a variety of scourges. The last part of the play makes overt allusions to pestilence. After Moses rejects Pharaoh's false oath that the Israelites can go free, Pharaoh asks one of his people, "Why, is there grievance grown again?" (314). One of the Egyptians answers: "Such powder, lord, upon us drive / That where it beats

I makes a blain" (314–5). The word "blain" means "boil" which implies the boils commonly associated with plague infection. Furthermore, the ash coming down recalls the idea that God showered the earth with plague rays in order to infect the air. Following these lines, another Egyptian states:

> Like mesels make it man and wife.
> Sithen are they hurt with hail and rain;
> Our vines in mountains may not thrive,
> So are they thrust and thunder-slain. (317–20)

"Mesels" implies leprosy, but could also refer to a rash, called a plague girdle, that was common to infected people. Herlihy explains that the plague girdle is "Petechiae, small crimson or livid spots, [that] appear on the patient's skin in severe cases" (22). Herlihy also finds medical doctors in Avignon between 1373 and 1388 who find "pustules which appeared in the groin, legs, head, arms, or shoulders. They were livid in color, and numerous enough to form a rash over large areas of the body. The common people, he tells us, called this rash the 'plague girdle' " (27). This rash may be what the playwright of *Moses and Pharaoh* is relating to measles.

Pharaoh realizes that this punishment is sent down by God; as one of the counselors states, "My lord, great pestilence / Is like full long to last" (345–6). Pharaoh replies, "Oh, comes that in our presence? / Then is our pride all passed" (347–8). Once again, a medieval author emphasizes the connection between pestilence and pride. Pharaoh is too prideful and does not realize until too late that Moses is relaying messages from God. Because of Pharaoh's pride, particularly because he thinks he can make false oaths concerning Jewish freedom, he is ravaged by the plague. The mentions of plague and the symptoms of infection are not only a memorial to the people of York who suffered through the plague's visitation; they are also a reminder of what brings plague about: pride and false oaths. Moreover, since York had been struck by a visitation of the plague during the time of the play's assumed creation, and since this visitation seemed to take children, it makes sense that the story about a man-made method of killing children should be connected to the divine epidemic.

Conclusions

The representations of pestilence in medieval literature are indeed varied and complex. Beidler writes,

> I do not feel, however, that we can understand the Pardoner or his *exemplum* if we overlook either the plague backdrop which Chaucer provided for the story or the evidence concerning medieval attitudes toward the plague. To overlook these is to be blind to important elements of incident, character, and theme. (265)

Lacking any knowledge of vector-borne diseases, people of the Middle Ages were left to conclude that the plague was a consequence of sinful behavior. The job of the medical, theological, and literary community was to interpret the meaning of the plague, the causes of God's anger and man's sin. Some of those answers centered on the idea that plague punished pride; other answers focused on the role of false oaths and cursing. While these sins were not new to the fourteenth century, what was new was a widely dispersed divine punishment for individual human sin. Therefore, in the early decades of infection, people ascribed the disease to general sins, like pride, because nearly everyone is guilty of these sins. Even though many individuals believed that sin brought about the plague, they also attempted to identify the natural causes of the disease, such as earthquakes and astrological alignments. Nevertheless, a natural cause for the plague did not preclude a divine, moral reason for its presence. God remained the First Mover and controller of the natural world.

Literary works provide readers with information about life changes that may help them to avoid plague. Many authors identified health regimens similar to those identified by the medical community. People were encouraged to moderate their drinking, eating, and exercise. Authors like Langland went as far as offering the medical belief that pestilence travels on the south wind and, therefore, avoidance of that wind would make sense. While much of this information no longer seems logical, this medical information was the most authoritative and current of its day. The literary work was simply passing that information on to the readers so that they could protect themselves from the ravages of plague.

Another aspect that literary works offered was reflection by which a reader could see his or her contribution to the continuation of the pestilence. In most cases, the authors discuss general characteristics and common social sins in order to demonstrate that each person contributes to God's anger and therefore to the continuation of the disease. Eventually the plague becomes so common that people begin to deal with it as a normal part of the human experience. Consequently, literary authors treat the disease more pragmatically. In other words, instead of seeing the disease as a representation of God's anger with man for his sins, literary authors begin to see the plague as part of a lived experience. They realize that not everyone is going to die from the disease, and the disease becomes as common as diarrhea, arthritis, and cancer. The disease, consequently, becomes part of normal experience. If one lives long enough, he or she will experience plague, either directly or indirectly. The next chapter will explore how the framework of the disease altered as people began to see this disease as part of human experience.

CHAPTER FIVE

Learning to Cope with Disease

Since bubonic plague recurred time and time again, people living in the fifteenth and sixteenth centuries eventually began to cope with the disease in a different way than their predecessors had. While fourteenth-century Europeans saw the plague as an unparalleled event, those in the fifteenth century recognized plague as a normal, albeit unfortunate, part of life. Hays explains:

> [B]y the fifteenth century the members of health boards gradually began acting on more clearly contagionist assumptions. Those assumptions led to more direct interference with both individuals and groups. Occasions that brought crowds together became suspect, and were thus objects of regulation: schools, church services, and—especially—the very religious processions that so many towns had sponsored to propitiate God's wrath. The movements of the suspiciously transitory classes—especially beggars, soldiers, and prostitutes—came under scrutiny. Boards of health also, in their attempt to stay informed, began recording the causes of death in their cities. The early censuses of death themselves contributed to changing conceptions of disease. (54)[1]

The changing conceptions of disease created a new discourse in which the individual became responsible for protecting himself or herself from disease. It became possible to avoid the contagion, and literature was one of the avenues by which the discourse about plague protection was disseminated.

Rather than examining the collective sins of the community and the possibility that this disease was linked to the apocalypse, literary authors focused more heavily on methods of diagnosis, cure, and treatment. In *The Impact of Plague on Tudor and Stuart England*, Paul Slack writes,

> If some published tracts emphasised God's hand in the origins and incidence of epidemics, others stressed their natural and predictable features

> and deduced that action could be taken against them. Individuals could act effectively by keeping their houses clean, avoiding sources of infection, burning the bedding and clothing of the sick and so on. The dangers of miasma and contagion could also be attacked, and potentially more successfully, by governments. Against miasma, fires might be lit in the streets and open and shallow graves could be more strictly controlled. Against infection, it should be possible to restrict movement of domestic animals—cats, dogs, and pigs—who might transmit disease from house to house. A whole programme of administrative activity and regulation could be built upon commonplace assumptions about plague. (45)

These commonplace assumptions find their way into literary works which try to disseminate the information to a more general audience.

In the previous chapter, I demonstrated that both Langland and Chaucer identified life regimens that medical doctors supported as a means to avoid plague. Nevertheless, disease transmission and methods of protection were not the primary concern for either author. Instead, these authors focused on the causes of the plague's existence. They wanted to identify the sin that made God so angry. In the sixteenth and seventeenth centuries, plague transmission and methods of protection become more important to literary authors than the interpretation of the meaning of plague. This change in focus can be demonstrative of a desire to take more control over the course of plague, to change it from an event with is completely controlled by God to one that has some human interaction. For example, in *A defensative against the plague*, a pamphlet published between March 25 and April 6, 1593, in England, Simon Kellwaye lists the possible causes of the disease. These causes include: the heat, the rain, decomposing bodies, filth, overcrowding, wearing clothing of the dead, and certain animals, such as pigs, dogs, cats, and weasels. All of these possible causes are natural, but near the end of the list of possible causes, Kellwaye writes, "But howsoever it doth come, let vs assure our selues that it is a just punishment of God layde vpon vs, for our manyfold sinnes and trangressions against his diuine Maiestie" (qtd. in Barrett vi). The sins are no longer a specific few, but many. More importantly, the causes of the disease are, for the most part, controllable. Slack writes, "Although God was the first cause of plague, however, he normally worked through secondary causes, 'by what constant course of order which he hath appointed unchangeable from the beginning'. This natural machinary could be studied and profitable lessons learned" (26). Unlike the belief in the cooperation of Saturn and Mars or the belief in pestilential earthquakes, many Renaissance beliefs about plague concern basic hygiene and vector transmissions via humans and animals. This practical information found its way into literary texts, and authors of those texts attempted to disseminate the new information to a wider audience.

There could be many reasons why the people of the sixteenth and seventeenth centuries interpreted the bubonic plague differently than prior generations. I believe the two greatest influences are that the disease no longer killed as many people when infection occurred and that the disease struck localized areas rather than entire countries or continents. Platt states,

> Nobody now denies the Black Death's status as a defining moment in late-medieval English history. But there are good reasons to tread cautiously all the same. It was famine, not plague, after 1349, that remained the biggest killer in the colder, wetter, and emptier northern countries. In those countries also, extended families lived on longer; while even in southern England, the Black Death's successor plagues may always have come second in population control to the growing practice of late marriage with fewer children. Gentry fell as often as they rose. More monks undoubtedly died of overweight or of liver conditions than ever succumbed to the plague. Many towns continued to prosper through a long recession which, for them at least, had seldom begun before the very end of the fourteenth century at the earliest. But with every reservation, one critical fact remains in place. England from 1400 was half-empty. (190)

The first pandemic of 1348–49 decimated the English population, but succeeding visitations rarely killed more than 10 to 15 percent of the population (Gottfried, *Black Death*, 131). As Platt argues, there were other diseases killing people that usurped plague as the King of Death. Consequently, plague became part of the fabric of life, and works of literature reflect a change from apocalyptic vision to practical methods of protection.

In the scholarly and historical works on bubonic plague, there is little said about the changing social attitudes toward the plague in fifteenth- and sixteenth-century England. Moreover, there is even less work done on literary authors who write about plague. John Lydgate (c.1370–c.1451) wrote two poems, "A Doctrine For Pestilence" and *A Dietary*, which were often printed separately, but are also found combined in the Lansdowne manuscript, which was reprinted by *Early English Text Society*. The "Doctrine" is 24 lines of poetry, and the *Dietary* is 143 lines. Because both works deal with a similar theme, namely how to protect one's health, I will deal with them, simply as a matter of convenience, as one complete poem. The poem offers the reader information about a physical and psychological health regimen to avoid illness. The easily memorizable poem uses iambic pentameter lines rhymed ababbcbc.

William Bullein (d.1576) is the second author I examine in relation to the changing social response to plague. In *A Dialogue Against the Feuer Pestilence*, Bullein provides a prose work that could be considered an estate satire as the characters come from various social positions. This work also provides information about the plague in order to protect readers from infection.

In order to approach the role of literature in plague discourse, one must first be reminded that fictional literature of the fifteenth and sixteenth centuries had a greater level of social importance than it enjoys now. Authors were generally not as well disposed to falsifying facts as they might be today. Consequently, authors could use their story to transmit accurate medical information to their readers. While the use of literature as a vehicle for fact or health information seems unlikely to our modern sensibilities, one must remember that even when our own medical doctors discuss accomplishments and discoveries, they fall back on narrative, on a form of literature, to transmit their information to others in an understandable fashion. Narratives can also be informative.

Only a few critics have examined the relationship between medicine and narrative. In *The Postmodern Condition*, Jean-François Lyotard argues that "scientific knowledge does not represent the totality of knowledge; it has always existed in addition to, and in competition and conflict with, another kind of knowledge, which I will call narrative" (7). Lyotard believes that modern scientific thought is caught in a paradox, for it "cannot know and make known that it is the true knowledge without resorting to the other, narrative, kind of knowledge, which from its point of view is no knowledge at all" (29). Instead, scientific knowledge employs a language of denotation, a language that inherently questions its own validity. Furthermore, since most non-scientists are used to the language of narrative and are unfamiliar with the language of science, denotation systematically separates the common reader from the scientist. Consequently, scientific knowledge becomes unattainable for the majority of people (Lyotard 32–33). In order to make scientific knowledge attainable for the majority of people, scientists rely on the narrative to explain their discovery. This narrative is at some level in conflict with the scientific language because, by nature of the allusive language it must employ, a narrative is partly untrue. But, as Lyotard rightly suggests, this conflict was not always the case for scientific knowledge. Before 1900, few questioned narrative as a truthful means of scientific transmission (Lyotard 24). Consequently, narrative, as well as other forms of literary transmission, was a viable means to communicate complex medical ideas to other individuals in a memorable way. Literature serves as a medium by which difficult scientific and medical information can be made accessible to the common person.

One needs only to look at the *Regimen Sanitatis Salernum* for the value of poetry in the medical field. The *Regimen* is a publication in Leonine verse from the medical school of Salerno. The work was translated into numerous languages and was expanded "three, four, and five times its length before again being reduced by critical research to its original length" (*School of Salernum* 17). More interesting for the early seventeenth century is that the long Latin poem was translated into English by John Harrington, Prince Henry's Tutor, and published in 1607. Harrington's translation uses rhymed heroic couplets, most likely because they are the easiest to commit to memory.

The narrative was a useful tool by which to disseminate medical information to the general population during epidemics. The narrative took many forms, one of which is the pamphlet. Slack speaks to the growing importance placed on the publication of medical tracts in the early modern period:

> [Assumptions about plague] are articulated most clearly for the historian . . . in the many printed medical tracts of the period which discuss plague and disease in general. Although often ostensibly written for the poor, these works were in fact handbooks for middle-class households and for unqualified medical practitioners in a society in which doctors were few. They thus expressed and influenced the views of the literate and articulate classes. But their contents and their popularity suggest that they also reflected some of the more pervasive assumptions and anxieties about disease in early modern England. (23)

The increase in the number of pamphlets about plague demonstrates that people were interested in learning about ways to avoid and cope with the disease. Moreover, literature was an important medium that enabled the medical and scientific information to be brought to a more general audience.

JOHN LYDGATE'S *DIETARY* AND "A DOCTRINE FOR PESTILENCE"

Lydgate's poem recalls many of the ideas about plague presented in the Middle Ages. Douglas Gray writes, "Lydgate's *Dietary* seems to have been one of the most popular of medieval English poems, at least with scribes and compilers of manuscripts. *The Index of Middle English Verse* and its *Supplement* list no fewer than fifty-five copies (Nos. 824, 1418), a number which is surpassed only by the *Pricke of Conscience* and the *Canterbury Tales*" (245). The poem's popularity seems to be derived from the practical information that this work gives the reader. The last three lines state the poem's purpose: "This receiht bouht is of non appotecarie, / Off Maister Antony, nor of Maister Hewe; / To all indifferent richest dietarie!" (21.166–68). The poem is not something that was purchased from or sold by doctors or pharmacists, but it was free to all readers to help them avoid illness.

The major difference between Lydgate's work and other works on illness is that Lydgate seems to have little interest in proving the divine cause of illness. While many readers of Lydgate would find it shocking that he does not moralize disease, he seems to have little interest in interpreting the meaning of illness as a divine or mystical means of communication. Instead he is interested in providing the most current medical information about avoiding the disease. While Gray believes that modern readers will find this "the dullest of medieval poems," he does recognize the important place that works like the *Dietary* occupied in the fifteenth century. Gray writes, "[I]n the fifteenth century there does seem to have been some sort of demand for these informative 'practical' verses; there are others on such unpromising subjects as bloodletting and the medicinal properties of leeks" (245). Gray would like to see Lydgate's "practical verse" as "proverbial;" however, the organization of the subject matter follows common academic medical structures of the six non-naturals, which are air, exercise and rest, sleep and waking, food and drink, repletion and excretion, and the passions or emotions.[2] Furthermore, we begin to see a shift in the community's interpretation of disease. By Lydgate's time in the fifteenth century, people were becoming more concerned with providing medical advice on how to protect each other than they were about finding the divine reason for illness. Lydgate does not seem to reject the idea that morality influences an individual's health, but he does seem to reject the idea that plague is a reflection of a single sin, that of pride or false oaths such as in the fourteenth century with Langland and Chaucer. For Lydgate, plague can be avoided through a series of psychological, moral, and physical adjustments.

The *Dietary* seems to be connected to the "Doctrine" by the discussion of melancholy in relation to the six non-naturals. In the "Doctrine" the six non-naturals are referenced in a reduced fashion; however, in the *Dietary*, Lydgate offers an expansion on each of the six non-naturals. Interestingly, the two works seem to be connected because in the middle of the *Dietary*, Lydgate states, "Fire at morwe & toward bed at eve, / Ageyn mystis blake & heir of pestilence" (17.129–30). This refrain of "mystis blake" is the ending lines of the three stanzas of the "Doctrine." Consequently, these two works seem to inform each other.

In both the "Doctrine" and the *Dietary*, Lydgate uses the six non-naturals to structure his poem. The passions and emotions are figured into the first three lines of the "Doctrine" where Lydgate advocates optimism. Lydgate writes, "Who will bee holle & kepe hym from sekenesse / And resiste the strok of pestilence, / Lat hym be glad, & voide al hevynesse" (1.1–3). According to Lydgate, one's psychological state influences one's health. The concept underlying the relationship between emotions or passions and illness is related to the idea of the humors. Each humor is connected to a psychological state, as our own adjectives sanguine, choleric, phlegmatic, and melancholic testify. If someone was thought to be exceptionally sad, he or she could be producing melancholy that could threaten his or her health.

The most famous work on melancholy is Robert Burton's *The Anatomy of Melancholy* (1628). While Burton's work is written nearly 200 years after Lydgate's poem, he relies on a host of medical experts from the Greco-Roman period through the sixteenth century to arrive at his definition and cause. Much of the medical knowledge Burton describes changed little over the centuries; therefore his work tends to be a storehouse of medical ideas about the body and disease that were common from the Middle Ages through the Early Modern Period. Concerning the causes of melancholy, Burton writes, "Fear & Sorrow are the true characters, and inseparable companions, of most melancholy" (149). Melancholy exists in a natural state in the body, but when it or other humors become burnt or scorched, melancholy becomes unnatural and leads one into a poor physical state (Burton 152–3). The humors may become burnt through a variety of metaphysical and physical methods, but one way is through emotions. Burton writes,

> For as the body works upon the mind, by his bad humours, troubling spirits, sending gross fumes into the brain, and so disturbing the soul, and all the faculties of it,
>
> *The body, clogged with yesterday's excess,*
> *Drags down the mind as well,* (Horace)
>
> with fear, sorrow, &c. which are ordinary symptoms of this disease: so, on the other side, the mind most effectually works upon the body, producing by his passions and perturbations miraculous alterations, as melancholy, despair, cruel disease, and sometimes death itself, insomuch, that is most true which Plato saith in his Charmides, all the mischeifs of the body proceed from the soul. (217–18, Latin translated by Dell and Jordon-Smith)

Burton sees a relationship between the body and the mind in which both can produce substances that influence melancholy. The body produces vapors that cloud the brain's functions, and the brain can produce melancholy in the body by focusing on negative emotions.

The relationship between emotional state and health is very important in the fifteenth century. While in the "Doctrine" Lydgate mentions gladness as a way to avoid the plague, in the *Dietary*, Lydgate moves beyond just telling his reader to avoid sad thoughts. He tells the reader to "keep welle thi-silf from incontynence" (2.13), and to do things in a temperate manner. Lydgate's advice is the same dietary regimen that Piers receives from Hunger in Langland's work. Lydgate makes his poem into a medical prescription; however, the medicine is for the most part a psychological state. Even when Lydgate appears to be writing physical prescriptions, the actual remedies are part of the psychological rather than physical realm. Lydgate writes:

> Ther be thre lechees consarue a mannys myht,
> First a glad hert, he carith lite or nouht,
> Temperat diet, holsom for every with,
> And best of all, for no thyng take no thouht.
>
> Care a-way is a good medycyne
> Digest afforn, preparat with gladnesse. (8–9. 61–66)

Lydgate is using a form common to medical manuscripts to provide a psychological prescription for his readers. To avoid illness, readers are supposed to remain happy and not think too seriously. In order to do this, Lydgate suggests, that they take "Care a-way" prepared with gladness; thus Lydgate offers the reader a prescription much as medical doctors do, but his prescription relies on emotional and psychological states, rather than actual plants and herbs. Nevertheless, his advice corresponds to common medical theories about the way the emotions influence one's humoral balance and, in turn, one's health.

Lydgate's prescriptions move beyond an individual psychological realm into a social realm. Like Chaucer's Pardoner, who seems to be suggesting that plague is caused by false oaths, Lydgate also offers the reader methods of social interaction under the guise of a dietary. Lydgate writes:

> Be clenly claad aftir thyn estat,
> Passe nat thi boundis, keep thi promys blive,
> With thre folks be nat at debate,
> First with thi bettir be war for to stryve,
> Ageyn thi felaw no quarell do contryve,
> With the soget to fihten it were shame,
> Wher[for] I counsel pursewe al thi lyve
> To live in pes & gete the a good name.

Lydgate emphasizes the importance of keeping one's word to others as well as keeping a clean house. He also states that the people should know their social place and know how to live within that framework. Lydgate offers the reader some sound advice: he or she should not quarrel with those who are better than him or her, and those who are socially inferior to the reader should not be fought with because it would be shameful. By following these rules, Lydgate states, one will live a good life because he or she will live in peace and have a good reputation. Adherence to social rules seems to affect one's health because it enables one to lead a happier life. The emphasis on social hierarchy and rules is designed to create happier individuals, which in turn creates a happier community that is relatively disease free. While this information seems markedly similar to that used by Langland and Chaucer, Lydgate draws little connection between these psychological and social rules and divine retribution. By Lydgate's time, illness seems to have changed from divine vengeance that kills entire communities to a disease that attacks those who are weakened by bad psychological outlooks and poor social relations.

One may be led to infer that since Lydgate is giving a psychological prescription for ways to avoid illness and plague, he may be mocking the medical community. This seems highly unlikely because other parts of the poem praise doctors and offer typical physical regimen changes. Lydgate writes:

> And yiff so be leechis doth the faile,
> Than take good heed to vse thynges thre,
> Temperate diet, temperate travaile,
> Nat melancholius for non adversite,
> Meeke in trouble, glad in pouerte,
> Riche with litel, content with suffisaunce,
> Never grucchyng, mery lik thi degre,
> Yiff phisik lak, make this thi gouernance. (13.97–104)

It may be possible to read the words "faile" and "lak" in the first and last lines as demonstrative of a growing impatience with the medical community. However, since Lydgate's advice follows the beliefs common to authoritative medical learning, it would seem unlikely that he is condemning medical knowledge. A different reading could be that "faile" and "lak" imply that doctors are unavailable. As we have seen in the previous chapters, authoritative medical professionals were available in larger urban environments, but in more rural areas there were fewer university-trained doctors. Consequently, other discourses, such as treatises on rural practices and penitential manuals, sometimes contained medical information meant to be passed on by those in charge. This poem seems to be providing similar practical information.

Lydgate also offers practical information about the air that one breathes. Like Langland's concern with the south-west wind, Lydgate advises his reader to "Smelle swote thyng[es] & for his deffence / walk in cleene heir, eschew[e] mystis blake" (l. 7–8). This idea is so important to Lydgate that he makes it a refrain for the first two stanzas. The avoidance of certain winds is also related to the production of melancholy: "Montanus will have tempestuous and rough air to be avoided, and all night air, and would not have them to walk abroad but in pleasant day" (Burton 209–10). Lydgate's advice to avoid the dark air could be related to either the medical idea that disease travels on the wetter southern wind or to the general idea that wet weather creates bad melancholy in an individual.

What is clearly related to official advice is the idea that one needs to avoid bad smells as a means of protection. For example, the famous English manuscript of John of Burgundy (c. 1365) also identifies wet air and bad smells as the cause of plague:

> In cold or rainy weather you should light fires in your chamber and in foggy or windy weather you should inhale aromatics every morning before leaving home: ambergris, musk, rosemary and similar things if you are rich; zedoary, cloves, nutmeg, mace, and similar things if you are poor ... and carry in the hand a ball of ambergris or other suitable aromatic. Later, on going to bed, shut the windows and burn juniper branches so that the smoke and scent fills the room. Or put four live coals in an earthenware vessel and sprinkle a little of the following powder on them and inhale the smoke through mouth and nostrils before going to sleep: take white frankincense, labdanum, storax, calaminth, and wood of aloes and grind them to a very fine powder. And do this as often as a foetid or bad odour can be detected in the air, and especially when the weather is foggy or the air tainted, and it can protect against the epidemic. (Horrox 186–87)

In Burgundy's treatise, one can see the emphasis placed on the dangers of moist air and bad smells. There was no concept that diseases could be carried on the air; instead the idea was that air that smelled bad or air that was damp adjusted the humoral balance, thereby bringing about more bad melancholy and, hence, sickness.

Besides concern about air, Lydgate also recommends dietary modifications. These too correspond to the medical community's advice to monitor food and drink. Lydgate writes, "Drynk good wyn & holsom meetis take" (1. 7). Later he recommends:

> Ete nat gret flessh for no greedynesse,
> And fro frutes hold thyn abstynence,
> Poletis & chekenys for ther tendirnesse
> Ete hem with sauce, and spar nat for dispence. (3. 17–20)

The emphasis on diet follows authoritative medical advice and is also connected to melancholy. Burton states, "The first of [the six non-naturals] is diet, which consists in meat and drink, and causes melancholy, as it offends in substance, or accidents, that is, quantity, quality, or like" (189). Red meats are believed to cause melancholy as are certain types of fowl; however, chicken is not banned in Burton's dietary (190–91). Burton also states that "a cup of wine is good physick . . . if it be moderately used" (194–95). Lydgate even uses an authoritative reference to his defense of wine as healthy:

> In thi drynkis put cleene sawge & rewe,
> Bothe be good & holsom of natur,
> And phisik seith, the rose flour-is dewe,
> And Ypocras recordith in scriptur
> Good wyn is holsom to euery creatur
> Take in mesur, with v. addiciouns,
> Strong, fressh, & colde, off tarage, & verdur
> Most commendid a-mong al naciouns. (6.41–8)

Other dietary advice Lydgate offers is "Levenyn bred . . . made of good whete flour (5. 33–4), sage and rue drinks (6.41), and wholesome wine (6.45).

Related to one's diet is another non-natural, repletion and excretion. While Lydgate does not mention anything about urinalysis, he does talk about proper times to eat and drink. In the "Doctrine," Lydgate writes, "With voide stomach outward the nat dresse" (2.1). To avoid the plague, one needs to avoid going out on an empty stomach and make sure not to overeat. The *Dietary* explains when are appropriate times to eat:

> Greedi souper & drynkyng late at eve
> Causith of fflewme gret superfluyte;
> Colre adust doth the stomak greve,
> Melancolik a froward gest, parde!
> Of mykil or litel cometh al infirmyte

Attween thes too for lak of governaunce,
Dryve out a mene, excesse or scarsete,
Set thi botaill vpon temeraunce. (10.73–80)

Once again, Lydgate emphasizes the relationship between melancholy and illness. If one eats too much or too little or eats and drinks too late, he or she produces more choler, thereby increasing the possibility for melancholy. Essentially those most interested in maintaining health should practice moderation: "Moderat diet ageyns al seekenessse, / Is best phisicien to mesur thyn entraile" (11. 87–88).

The information that Lydgate offers to his reader fits common medical knowledge. Burton declares, "There is not so much harm proceeding from the substance itself or meat, and quality of it, in ill dressing and preparing, as there is from the quantity, disorder of time and place, unseasonable use of it, intemperance, overmuch or overlittle taking of it" (196). Not only does Lydgate mention that one should eat not too much or too little and be temperate, but he also underscores that food should be eaten in its season. Lydgate states: "Temperat diet kyndly digestioun / . . . Naturall appetite abydyng his sesoun, / Foode accordyng to the complexioun" (12. 90–3). If one practices these methods, both Lydgate and Burton believe that he or she will not create more melancholy and thereby avoid illness: "that froward maladie" (Lydgate 12. 96).

Sleeping and waking is also an important part of the regimen Lydgate advises. In the "Doctrine," Lydgate tells his reader to rise early with a fire (2.10), but then states, "The morwe sleep, callid gyldene in sentence, / Gretly helpith aygeen the mystis blake" (3.24). This seems to be a conflict in regimen. Most doctors advised a moderate hour to rise, but if we look at ways to avoid melancholy, we find that sleeping in the morning was a good prophylactic. Burton writes: "It is a received opinion, that a melancholy man cannot sleep over-much; excessive sleep is good, as an only antidote, and nothing offends them more, or causeth this malady sooner, than waking" (216). Lydgate's recommendation to rise early seems to be connected to the fire and the purity of the air. The fire, a good smell, will keep the pestilence away. However, in the second recommendation to sleep late, Lydgate is recalling the idea that morning sleep keeps away melancholy, thereby also protecting the body from illness. In the *Dietary*, Lydgate insists that the reader should be "[g]lad toward bedde and at morwe" (4.31), "in especial flee meridan sleep," (5.40), and "after mete bewar, make no sleepe (19. 145). Lydgate is following the general medical belief that happy thoughts can help one's health and that one should avoid afternoon naps and sleeping after one eats. All of these activities can be altered for better health. Burton explains, "Or if [sleep] be used in the day time, upon a full stomack . . . such sleep prepares the body, as one observes, to many perilous diseases" (217). The daytime nap and sleeping on a full stomach are dangerous habits. The information that Lydgate relates to the reader corresponds to common medical theories about the time to rise and when to sleep so as to avoid increased melancholy.

Finally, Lydgate offers advice on how someone should exercise or work. In the "Doctrine", Lydgate states that one should "walk in cleene air, … delite in gardeyns for ther gret swetnesse" (1–2. 8–11). This advice can be seen in relation to two of the non-naturals: air and exercise. Lydgate may not be referring to a low-impact walking regimen because these lines could simply be related to pleasing air. However, when one looks at the "Dietary," Lydgate's implied meaning become obvious: "And eschew excesse of labour / Walk in gardeyns sote of ther savour" (5. 36–7). Gardens give people a way to smell fragrances that are appealing and healthy, but the connection to labor links this advice to the non-natural category of exercise and work. Burton argues for a moderate exercise and work regimen: "Nothing better than exercise (if opportunely used) for the preservation of the body: nothing so bad, if it be unseasonable, violent, or overmuch" (210). Lydgate connects labor to walking in gardens for the sweet smell of the flowers. The activities of labor and exercise are ways to keep away melancholy and, in turn, disease.

The health regimen Lydgate offers to avoid plague in the "Doctrine" is very similar to the ways to avoid general illness as prescribed in the *Dietary*. Consequently, the two works were joined together, at least in this one manuscript. In other words, plague is treated as commonly as melancholy or general illness. The regimen that one uses for plague is the same that one uses to keep oneself healthy. Lydgate's work finds no mystical or divine meaning for the plague, which is especially odd since Lydgate was a monk. There is not even a theory as to how the disease originated. The only religious advice Lydgate offers the reader in the *Dietary* consists of general guidelines:

> First at thi risyng to God do reverence,
> Visite the poore with enteer diligence,
> On al nedy have pite & compassioun,
> And God shall sende the grace & influence
> The tenchrece, & thi possessioun (17. 132–36).

This sentiment is far from Langland's interpretation of plague and far from an apocalyptic vision of illness. At least for Lydgate, pestilence has changed from being a means of divine communication between man and God to a common aspect of illness. There is no attempt to single out the meaning of the plague any more than there is to single out the meaning of a toothache. Plague has become part of the medical warp and the literary weft of the social web rather than an apocalyptic sign.

William Bullein's *Dialogue Against the Fever Pestilence*

Like Lydgate's "Dietary," William Bullein's *Dialogue Against the Fever Pestilence* (1564) was a very popular work that has not received the critical attention it deserves, although Slack believes the work to be '[p]erhaps the most effective literary treatment of [plague] issues" (41). Related to Anne Boleyn, Bullein was a doctor and a cleric who was born sometime "between 1520 and 1530 and died in 1575/6" (McCutcheon 341). He "serv[ed] as rector of Blaxhall, Suffolk in 1550, and subsequently practic[ed] as a doctor, first in the north of England and later in London, where he was living by 1560" (McCutcheon 341). Bullein was an ardent defender of Protestantism, but his work speaks to secular as well as theological ideas about disease. Elizabeth McCutcheon writes,

> The *Dialogue* has as its immediate context an outbreak of bubonic plague in London in June, 1563, made worse 'by the return of Elizabeth's already infected troops from her ill-fated attack on Le Havre in August of the same year': at least 18,000 people died, according to one source, 20,000 (close to a quarter of London's population), according to another. (341)

The *Dialogue*, however, does not reveal an apocalyptic vision of the plague's visitation. Instead, it offers practical medical advice designed to protect an individual from infection as well as a satire about avarice in certain social circles.

It is difficult to see a clear method of organization for Bullein's work, but that does not mean that one is absent. In the early part of the book, Bullein imagines a doctor, apothecary, and patient who discourse on ways to preserve one's life in the face of pestilence. The apothecary assumes that the patient will die, and both the doctor and the apothecary abandon him before the end. Bullein then introduces the reader to a citizen, his wife, and their servant. In the end, the wife remains in hiding and the servant abandons him when Death rides upon the citizen and announces that it is time to die. The citizen is left only with a theologian who offers him absolution and prayer to be said at the time of death. It seems that Bullein is attempting to write a work that helps people to prepare for both pestilence and death, an *ars moriendi*. What is markedly different about this work from those of the Middle Ages is the fact that plague is not seen as a precursor of Apocalypse, but as a part of everyday life.

Bullein's *Dialogue* deals with a variety of subjects and themes; however, the one most important to this study is his conception and construction of plague. In the *Dialogue*, only two characters, Antonius and Civis, become infected with plague. Each character receives information from a medical doctor, but only one is able to receive help from a priest. Neither character recovers from the disease, so it is difficult to say which information was most beneficial. Critics of the *Dialogue* have found it to be chaotic and unwieldy. McCutcheon speaks about the critical reception of the *Dialogue*:

> According to C. S. Lewis, for example, Bullein "was trying to do too many things at once. He wanted to write prescriptions against the Plague, satire

> against usurers, satire against lawyers, a Protestant tract, a catalogue of Emblems, and a Dance of Death." In fact, Lewis's list is not complete: the *Dialogue* includes a garden of the muses, an anthology of English poetry, a philosophical discourse on the nature of the soul, beast fables, and an *ars moriendi* and a consolation in time of death, as well as a utopia. (343)

The list of topics that Bullein attempts to handle is indeed overwhelming, but Bullein recognizes the book's diversity when he compares his work to a house that has a variety of decorative schemes. Bullein writes, "Therefore, the diuersitie or varietie of pleasaunte colours dooe grace and beautifie the same through the settyng forth of sondrie shapes: and as it were to compell the commers in to beholde the whole worke" (1).[3] It is nearly impossible for any critic to behold the whole work.[4] Some critics, like Herbert Wright, see the *Dialogue* as an eloquent statement "on the fading of beauty and the frailty of man" (42). Others, like Albert Baugh, read Bullein's work as a witty "collection of tall tales with a framing narrative" (413). Sections of the work are alternately serious and flippant, didactic and satiric, and it is nearly impossible to provide one generic rubric or theme for the work. Finally, William Boring sees the work as demonstrative of the anti-Papist tendencies of the Protestant reformation. Boring believes that the "dominant unifying note in the *Dialogue* [is] . . . that the Church *is* a plague, a danger to men's souls as surely as the disease is a danger to their bodies" (40).

It is difficult to discuss the meaning of the work as a whole, and most critics have difficulty merely identifying its genre. Since it is written as a dialogue, some critics have chosen to compare it to other dramatic works. For example, *The Cambridge History of English Literature* describes the work as a "drama of death. . . which reaches nearly every abuse of the age" (Ward 3. 108–09). One of the abuses of the Tudor age was avarice, and O. J. Campbell believes that Ben Jonson may be indebted to Bullein's work for part of the plot of *Volpone* (18–19). Boring, however, is the only critic to examine drama as a possible generic framework for Bullein's work. Boring reads Bullein's work as participating in the genre of morality plays, such as *Everyman*, where the characters reflect common social types. Boring writes that the work relies on "variations on the theme of *De contemptu mundi*" (40).

McCutcheon has done one of the most detailed genre studies of Bullein's work, and she uses the recent study by Jacqueline Proust, who sees the *Dialogue* as "divide[d] into two 'acts,' one in London, one on the road" (qtd. in McCutcheon 345). This division may remind some readers of Chaucer's *Canterbury Tales*, a work that has also confounded critics as to genre. McCutcheon sees this division as a problem because it "leav[es] us with a distorted sense of the relationship of one part of the work to another and undervalues its thematic and formal variety and its fascination with ideas and attitudes" (345). McCutcheon places the dialogue in the genre of a Menippean satire, or anatomy. Menippean satire is "framed by a loose narrative story" and "frequently feature[s] banqueting scenes or other settings in which extended and ridiculous debates take place. Far from being fully developed characters, the debaters are often little more than caricatures who merely serve to represent the ideas they expound" (Murfin and Ray 210). Most critics seem to agree that the *Dialogue* is a form of Menippean satire. Eugene Kirk also includes the *Dialogue* in a catalogue of Menippean satires, but he characterizes it as an "apocalyptic Lucianism" (qtd. in McCutcheon 345). The problem with this definition is that the *Dialogue* does not have an apocalypse. McCutcheon writes, "[T]he idea of judgment is doubly relevant, its application simultaneously satiric and spiritual. Yet the world as a whole does not come to an end, despite Roger's foreboding: 'I think the daie of Dome is at hande' (p.78)" (345). The world does not end in an apocalyptic vision here because the social interpretation of the meaning of plague has changed. It is not the end of the world; instead plague is something to deal with and attempt to live through. It provides the reader with an anatomy of suffering. In this reading, the *Dialogue* does, to paraphrase Lewis, mirror life (292).

McCutcheon chooses anatomy as the genre Bullein is writing in, and she offers Northrop Frye's definition of anatomy as

> 'a loose-jointed narrative form' that parodies and echoes countless other works and 'deals less with people as such than with mental attitudes.' A high energy work and, often, an 'encyclopaedic farrago' . . . the anatomy combines fantasy with morality, at its most concentrated present 'a vision of the world in terms of a single intellectual pattern.' (347)[5]

McCutcheon believes that the single unifying pattern Bullein is displaying is "the nature of humankind, both individually and corporeally" (348). While I think McCutcheon is correct in her assessment of genre, I also think one cannot ignore the title of Bullein's work, *A Dialogue Against the Fever Pestilence*. The work is a dialogue not simply about the nature of humankind, but about the nature of human kind when faced with plague. More importantly, it is not apocalyptic because the dialogue is *against* the *fever* of plague. In other words, the dialogue is actively responding to this disease for it addresses a symptom of plague, not the plague itself. Inherent in this title is the fact that the disease does not overcome the body. Rather the body is in the process of fighting it. The fever symbolizes the fight the body has in relation to the plague. Furthermore, this fight or fever is not simply physical but also spiritual. Just as the body burns from plague, so can the soul burn from sin. Consequently, it is not unusual to have both medical information about cures for the plague as well as spiritual advice to assist the soul in the event of death, especially from a writer who was both a clerk and a doctor.

The perceived lack of organization of Bullein's work springs from his attempt to unify his spiritual and physical worlds. Boring laments: "By now the reader has certainly perceived the structureless and episodic quality of the

Dialogue. Perhaps Bullein, in haste, simply wished to string together his religious, moral, and medical advice with no true attempt at dramatic unity" (37). The anatomy of the work rests on the changes the individual can make to protect himself or herself corporeally from plague and spiritually to prepare for death.

Bullein opens his work by discussing the reason for his writing in both the dedicatory epistle to Edward Barrette of Belhous and the introduction to the reader. In both of these introductory sections, one can see Bullein's attempt to unify the theological and medical worlds. In the epistle, Bullein writes:

> I have also not forgotten the shamfull syn which raigneth in this worlde called ingratitude, which linially came from the loines of that false vilain Judas, neither the sicopantes, gnatoes, liars, and flatters of this worlde, the verie poison of the soule. Oh better, saieth Salomon, is the woundes of the frend then the kisses of the flatterer. Further, how many meanes maie be vsed againste the Pestilence, as good aire, diete, medicines accordingly: the which, if it do not preuaile, then cometh on the merciles power of deth ouer all flesh. (1–2. 21–25, 1–4)

Clearly, Bullein sees a unified world in which both theological and medical information plays a role in saving people from the ravages of plague. For Bullein, the plague has been caused by those who are not true to their word—by flatterers—but that information does not prevent one from preparing for and avoiding the disease. It is for this latter reason that Bullein offers his reader very practical medical information.

The *Dialogue* represents a change in the social interpretation of the disease. No longer is the disease seen as part of the Apocalypse; instead, pestilence becomes part of a lived experience or a local corrector. Like the epistle, the introduction to the reader demonstrates a unity among medicine and theology, disease and sin. What is different between the epistle and the introduction is that the latter contains a clear statement about the social benefits of his information. Bullein writes, "When thei are touched by the fearfull stroke of the Pestilence of their nexte neighbour, or els in their owne familie, then thei use Medicines, flie the Airs, &c. Which indeede are verie good meanes, and not against Gods woorde so to doe" (3. 7–11). The intersection of medicine and theology is clearly articulated in Bullein's opening address to the reader. Medicine is simply a tool of man that God approves of, and Bullein's work is dedicated to providing the reader with medical information with which he or she can protect himself or herself as well as family members. Bullein also describes other religious actions people choose to do during plague time, including "sodaine deuotion" and "refuse[d] grace" (3. 11–14). Like Boccaccio's opening to *The Decameron* in which the faithful and the faithless are both described, Bullein also describes human responses to plague that vary from devotion to rejection. Bullein hopes that the reader will take the information from the book "in good parte" (3.21), thereby learning the proper way to protect against plague and prepare for death.

While Bullein's description may remind a reader of Boccaccio's list in "The First Day," the texts differ in that, for Bullein, pestilence reminds humans of the preciousness of life and the need for devotion to God. Boccaccio's list on the other hand is more objective, much like a report of traumatic events with little interpretation. The plague Bullein describes appears cyclical and localized. The cyclical nature of the plague is demonstrated by the idea that humans experience periods of prosperity in which they forget their neighbors. Pestilence reminds humans that they are connected both to other humans and to God. By Bullein's time, plague rarely decimated whole regions. Rather, it affected a town or city; therefore, the occurrence of plague was seen on a local rather than global level. These changes in the social interpretation of plague are important to understanding Bullein's characters and their actions.

In relation to plague, the *Dialogue* has two main characters, Antonius and Civis, both of whom die from plague. However, each character deals with plague differently. The *Dialogue* opens by introducing us to three characters, Mendicus, Civis, and Uxor. Mendicus begins by praising Civis and Uxor and praying that "oure dere Leddie Shidle and Defende you from this Pest" (5). Civis can be read as well-off city dweller, and his actions demonstrate that he and his wife are upstanding Christians. After Mendicus recites part of the Lord's Prayer, Civis declares the prayer to be reverently spoken and orders his wife to "giue the poore man somethyng to his dinner" (5). The wife, on the other hand, wants to hear the Lord's Prayer done "better before I giue hym any thing" (3). Civis chastises her by saying, "What a reconyng is this! Dame, doe as I commaunde you; he is poore; we haue plentie; he is verie poore and hongrie; therefore dispatche hym a gods name, and let him go" (3). The actions of Civis and Uxor reflect the problems Bullein poses in the introduction to the reader. During prosperous times, wealthy citizens forget their duties to people in need, and the people in need forget their devotion to God. Thus, Civis corrects his wife for not wanting to give the friar any food, but the wife corrects the friar for not doing the Lord's Prayer justice. It is difficult to assess whether the prayer was done justice, for Civis stops Mendicus before he can complete the prayer. Obviously, Civis is satisfied, but his wife is not. Bullein's *Dialogue* is framed by the concept of charity, which Uxor seems to lack. Plague forces people to be more charitable to one another because they need each other to survive.

The framework speaks to common social ideas about the body and the soul. The civic relationship men have with each other provides material charity which is the staple of life that the body needs in order to survive. The master of the body within this framework is the medical doctor who provides men with an understanding of the effects and causes of plague. But when the body can no longer be sustained, one needs to be concerned about the soul, and that is healed by a priest. Neither approach to disease is seen as evil or wrong, but simply necessary at certain points in one's life. Since Bullein was both a doctor and a clerk, this worldview should not be surprising, but it does represent a change in the way plague infection was being treated by the early sixteenth century.

The change in the social interpretation of plague is made clearest by Civis's response when Mendicus asks him why he has not fled the plague. Civis explains that he has sent his children away because

> youth are apte to take the Plague. And, further, parentes are more naturall to their children then children to their fathers and mothers. Nature dooeth descende, but not ascende. Also if the citezen should depart when the Plague dooe come, then there should not onely be no Plague in the Citie, but also the Citie should be voide and emptie for lacke of inhabitauntes therein, therefore Goddes will be doen among his people. I doe not intende to flee; notwithstandyng, I praie God of his mercie deliver us from this Plague, for if it doe continewe, God knowthe it will not onely take awaie a number of poore people, but many wealthie and lustie Marchauntes also. (8–9)

Civis clearly sees plague as being divinely sent and sanctioned; however, it is also only present for a limited time. He can send his children away in order to protect them because he knows that the plague will eventually abate. Slack finds that the protection of wives and children was quite common to civic authorities: "For most men the impulse to preserve self and family necessarily triumphed over other loyalties and obligations. . . . [S]ome magistrates and ministers obeyed the call of duty and stayed in infected towns, but they sent away their wives and children first; and there were more who left with their families" (20). Carmichael also notes, "Several researchers have pointed to a growing concern for the health and welfare of children, a concern that was reflected in a boom of hospitals and foundling homes farther from the end of the fourteenth century. What Herlihy has called a 'new concern for the survival of children' was fairly widespread in French and Italian cities of the fifteenth century" (52). Evidently Uxor and Civis demonstrate a similar concern for the welfare of their children as they have moved them from areas of infection to an area that is potentially healthier. Civis's logic seems to suggest that this type of flight from cities is good because it fits the divine purpose for plague. If plague is meant to make people like Civis and Uxor more charitable and devoted, then if innocent children flee, there will be no uncharitable people left for God to correct; therefore, the plague will end.

The ability to avoid the plague creates other fears in the lives of fifteenth- and sixteenth-century people. In *The Black Death and the Middle East*, Michael Dols identifies the major difference between the interpretations of bubonic plague in the Orient and Occident. For the Orient, plague was seen as a common disaster; flight from a disease sent by God to punish collective sin was seen as itself a sin (297–300). The Occident, on the other hand, saw the disease in relation to individual sin and the apocalypse and, therefore, Christians advocated flight from plague-infected cities (300).

In Bullein's work there seems to be a shift from the interpretation of plague as a Christian apocalyptic punishment to one of a temporary and limited punishment. Civis is worried that he may sin more by attempting to flee God's punishment than if he stayed and dealt with whatever God may bring. Uxor coaxes that they should both flee "and return merely home again when the Plague is paste, and the Dogge daies ended" (56). Civis is not convinced that flight is divinely approved, and he asks, "What is our life? It is a vapour that appeareth for a little tyme, and afterward vanishe awaie ... and if it please God wee will bothe departe and retourne againe at his good wille and pleasure, for wee are in his handes whether so euer wee doe go" (56–7). It appears that Civis acknowledges a temporary divine punishment rather than imagining an apocalyptic punishment. Both Civis and Uxor are in the hands of God, but this plague is not seen as the end of the world. Rather, it is seen as part of God's localized plan.

Mendicus's response to Civis also demonstrates a change in social interpretation of the disease. Mendicus states,

> If such plague doe ensue it is no greate losse. For, firste, it shall not onely deliuer the miserable poore man, woman, and barnes from hurte and carefulnesse into a better worlde, but ause cutte of many coueteous vsuers, which bee like fat vncleene swine, which gooe neuer good vntill thei come to the dishe, but wroote out euery plante that thei can come by; and like vnto greate stinkyng mucle medin hilles, which neuer doe pleasure vnto the Lande or grounde vntill their heapes are caste abroade to the profites of many, whiche are kepte neither to their owne comfortes nor others, but onely in beheading them; like vnto cruel Dogges liyng in a Maunger, neither eatyng the Haye them selues ne sufferyng the Horse to fee thereof hymself. And in sike plague we pure people haue muccle gud. Their loss is our lucke; when thei doe become naked, we then are clethed againste their willes; with thei dooles and almose we are reliued; their sickness is our health, their death our life. (9)

The Mendicant sees plague as a benefit to both to the poor and pure. If the plague strikes the poor, it offers them a release from a painful worldly life, as in the interpretation of the death of lepers as merciful. The plague also corrects those individuals who do not offer charity to the less fortunate. Through God's corrective, the poor can be taken care of against the wishes of those guilty of usury. Finally, plague is a good event for those who are morally pure, because the good gain from the death of the sinful. Plague, once again, is a social corrector, but it is not interpreted as an apocalypse. Plague helps the poor to live better lives, and it corrects man's relationship to man. Furthermore, plague is associated with the poor, a common connection for epidemic diseases. Hays explains, "[B]y the seventeenth century English opinion saw plague as a disease of the poorer urban districts, a social problem associated with poverty and disorder" (57). Even in the sixteenth century, writers were starting to connect the disease to the lower classes, in this case the poor.

What seems to be most problematic for readers of Bullein is the idea that one can both protect oneself against plague and prepare for his or her death. A modern comparison would be with cancer. Many of us desire new medical information about ways to avoid certain forms of cancer, such as colon and lung cancers, through lifestyle modifications. This does not preclude another groups of writers from explaining ways to fight against cancer once one is diagnosed with it or from offering advice on how to prepare for one's death. Bullein offers similar information to his reader. The only difference is that Bullein wants to give his reader both medical and spiritual advice under one title. In other words, he prepares his reader for *all* stages of the disease, from those uninfected to those infected.

The medical information Bullein offers is clearly academic and authoritative. However, he also critiques the effectiveness of academic medicine that excludes theology. Medicus, one of the characters of the dialogue, has an extended conversation with Antonius, a patient of Medicus who is extremely old. Medicus's apothecary, Crispine, demonstrates the relationship between doctors and apothecaries in the sixteenth century as well as a growing feeling that the medical community is taking advantage of the sick. As Medicus examines Antonius, Crispine states, "I will departe: his talke doeth so much trouble mee; mee thinke he doeth wounde my conscience. Also I will home, and caste awaie a great number of rotten drugs wherewith I haue gotten muche money in deceiuyng the people" (27). Medicus responds to Crispine, "The vicar of S. Fooles be your ghostly father. Are you so wise? Tary still with mee; let hym paie for your rotten drugs, for I may saye to you that he is almost rotten alreadie hymself; me think your conscience is to much spiced with sodaine deuotion" (27). Bullein is critically examining the medical community in which the doctor and the apothecary are in a financial relationship with each other. Doctors were often professionally tied to apothecaries, and this passage gives us a rare look at how these relationships worked. More importantly, medical knowledge does not seem to be questioned in Bullein's work, but rather the characters that employ that knowledge are ineffective. For instance, it is not that the herbs are bad medicine, but that they are rotten produce. Moreover, when the apothecary tries to mend his ways, the doctor is the one who prevents him. The doctor is not incompetent in his medical knowledge; rather he is spiritually incompetent. Medicus and Crispine can be read as foils for Antonius and Civis in that Medicus and Antonius both believe that the way to salvation is through the medical arts.[6] However, Crispine and Civis see medicine as limited, and the addition of theology as a social practice makes salvation possible.

Antonius serves as a means for Medicus to expound on different types of ailments and cures, all of which appear to be medically sound. Antonius asks the doctor questions about the humoral makeup of the body in relationship to the elements and the nature of the human soul. In this part of the dialogue, the reader finds out that Medicus is not spiritually schooled. Medicus states, "I professed to followe *Aristotle*, but my meanyng was that I credite not the Bible matters; I am no Diuine, I finde no reasons there for my tourne, they are to harde thynges for me; I commende them to *Darbel* and *Duns*, &c." (32). The doctor's lack of spiritual information does not jeopardize his knowledge of physical illness or disease. It does however point to an increasingly secular field of expertise that has fewer ties with church teaching. These fewer ties to church teaching, at least in Bullein's work, appear to hurt his effectiveness as a doctor, since his lack of spirituality seems connected to his desire to rob his patient through his apothecary.

After Mendicus discourses on the nature of the body and soul, Antonius wants Medicus to provide information about plague. The next five-hundred-and-fourteen lines focus on plague. Through Antonius's questions, Medicus produces a plague discourse which examines the disease's transmission, portents, and remedies. All of the information that Medicus gives Antonius is medically sound for the time period. Medicus begins by describing how the plague is transmitted through the air: "Pestilent feuer, saieth Hypocrates, is in two partes considered; the first is common to euery man by the corruption of the ayre; The second is priuate or particular to some men through euill diete, repletion, which bringeth putrification, and finally mortification" (36). We learn from the doctor that protection from the plague requires one to modify the air one breathes as well as the food one eats.

The doctor continues by describing the types of air that transmit plague and the mechanism by which infection is accomplished. Medicus says,

> When there doth come a sodaine alteration or change in the qualitie of water from Colde to heate, transmutation from sweetnesse to stincke, as it chaunceth in waters through corrupted mixture of putrified vapours infectyng bothe ayre and water, which of their owne simplicitie are cleane, but through euill mixture are poysoned; or when stronge Windes doe carrie pestilent fume or vapours from stinkyng places to the cleane partes, as bodies dead of the Plague vnburied, Or mortalitie in battaile, death of cattel, rotten Fennes, commyng sodainly by the impression of aire, creepyng to the harte, corruptyng the spirites, this is a dispersed Pestilence by the inspiration of the ayre. (36–37)

Bullein describes two types of smells that create plague, natural and human. The natural plague comes by winds passing over places that stink and picking up the infection and bringing the infection to places of habitation. The second type of infection has human agency as men do not practice proper hygienic methods, such as proper burial, or disposal of dead in war, or disposal of livestock. From Bullein's description of the causes of plague, the reader learns that people should be conscious of the types of air they are surrounded by and try to avoid bad smelling air as much as possible. The avoidance of foul-smelling air is believed by the academic medical community to be a deterrent and prevention of plague. Bullein's prescription can be read as an attempt to disseminate those means of protection to the readers of his work.

Bullein's Medicus also explains the season when the disease is most prevalent and the omens of the coming of the disease. The Medicus explains that Harvest season is the most dangerous and spring is the least, "and in the tyme of sundrie chaunge of windes, when the weather is hotte and moyste" (37). Like most of Bullein's contemporaries, he believes that the stars portend plague as do "eclipses of the Sunne and Moone" (37). Bullein also has other signs besides astrological ones, such as "when birdes do forsake their egges, flies or thinges bredyng vnder the ground do flie high by swarmens into the ayre, or death of fish or cattell, or any dearth goyng before" (38). Portents of impending plague are important especially if one is advocating flight, as Bullein does often. Once again, Bullein is preparing his reader with the information necessary to avoid plague.

Bullein's work also demonstrates a shifting interpretation about those most likely to become infected. In later periods, plague was often linked to the poor and filthy, and Bullein's work demonstrates that beliefs about the poor and unclean as carriers was a medical as well as social belief. Medicus states,

> Moste chiefly to theim vnder the place infected, then to sluttishe, beastly people, that keepe their houses and lodynges vncleane, their meate, drinke, and clothyng most noysome, their laboure and trauaile immoderate; or to theim which lacke prouident wisedome to preuente the same by good diete, ayre, medicine, &c.; or to the bodies hotte and moyste; and these bodies do infect other cleane bodies, and whereas many people doe dwell on heapes together, as *Auecen* saith, *Et communicat multitudine homimum.* (37)

Bullein implies two specific ideas in this passage. The first is that cleanliness of domestic living space is important in preventing plague. Carmichael states, "Both malnutrition and poor sanitation suffuse this picture of fifteenth-century urban mortality" (58). According to Bullein, sufferers of plague are those that live in "heapes" together; ones that could be guilty of malnutrition and poor sanitation. Carmichael concludes,

> Whether [the deaths] were truly due to *Y. pestis*, totally or in minor part, mattered little to those whose 'experience' of 'plague' was framed and shaped by these urban epidemics. The conclusion a Florentine observer could have drawn by the mid-fifteenth century was that plague was usually contagious and that it was predominantly a disease of the poor (89).

It would appear from Bullein's work that the same sentiment found in Florence was also present in London. Bullein's work demonstrates an alteration in perspectives about the plague from a disease that affected all social classes to one that affected only the poor, perhaps since the wealthy often had more opportunities to flee the plague.[7]

After Medicus answers Antonius's questions regarding the disease's transmission, signs, and symptoms, Antonius then asks Medicus if the doctor could offer defenses against infection. The medical information that Medicus gives Antonius is thorough and complete. Medicus first analyzes the six non-naturals as they influence plague (39–40). Antonius then asks Medicus what the treatment should be for someone who gets the plague. Medicus states that the person should be helped if he or she purges and then is bled, depending on his or her humoral makeup. (40–41). Antonius then asks about how to bleed and what types of medications are good for those infected. Medicus responds with a host of answers, including six prescriptions to be used by people suffering from the effect of bubonic plague (41–44). After discussing the early signs of infection including fever, buboes, unequal pulse, and stinking urine, Antonius feels that Medicus has "shewed more perilles then helpes" (46). Antonius then asks for "any remedies," to which Medicus responds that he has "rehearsed" this information before, but will do so again. This time Medicus offers one-hundred-and-thirty-eight lines of text that summarize and add to the information already given. In this text, he offers new recipes, powders, and perfumes for dealing with plague, but his information follows the general principles of the six non-naturals. Evidently Bullein wants his reader to learn from this information and to be able both to protect himself or herself from plague infection and to attempt cures when infection occurs.

The ending of Medicus's discourse is problematic because it appears that all this medical information is of no use to Antonius. Antonius responds to Medicus's request to remember well this information: "I warrant you I haue noted it well; and though it helpe not me, yet I trust it shall doe good to others when I am gone" (50). This statement could be read in a variety of ways. One possibility is that Antonius, and in turn Bullein, is mocking authoritative medical knowledge for being of little use. Indeed, Medicus is not at all moral or religious, and Bullein could be satirizing the entire profession and corpus of learning. However, it could also be that Antonius feels that he is too old to be worried about being infected by the plague but will pass the information onto other people. One must remember that Antonius is suffering from sleeping problems and not plague, at least at this moment. The major cause of his sleeping problems lies in dreams in which he "heare many ragged and sicke people crie vengeaunce on me, and men in prison also, that said I had undoen them to inriche myself" (27). As a way to alleviate Antonius's fear about using people, Medicus has a surgeon, Wise, bleed Antonius and comment how noble a heart the patient has and how his worst trouble is behind (28). Medicus may be giving Antonius all this information about plague so that Antonius can help others with advice and thereby feel as if he served his fellow human beings suffering from plague. However, once Antonius is gone, the medical information from Medicus will also disappear because this information is transmitted orally.

Bullein also constructs a textual tradition wherein Medicus passes his knowledge to Crispine, the apothecary, who asks for some recipes for plague that he "will write them, and putte them in my booke at home" (52). Medicus proceeds to give the apothecary a variety of cures, including two perfumes, one powder, and two cordials (54–55). The cures Medicus gives are in Latin, not in the vernacular, which seems to suggest that medical recipes in Latin are more authoritative than in the vernacular. Latin gives the prescriptions a certain value, since they are written in the language of medicine. Furthermore, the use of Latin for the prescriptions precludes illiterate individuals from using those medicines. Only those who knew Latin or could get someone to translate it for them would be able to use the prescriptions listed. Bullein put the general regimen that doctors advocated to protect against plague into the vernacular to make it available to wider population in order to save the greatest number of people. The prescriptions, on the other hand, remain in Latin, which speaks both to their authority as medically authored cures and to a social hierarchy that knows Latin, but keeps the knowledge much to itself.

The apothecary thanks Medicus for his help, and prays to God that He will "make the ayre, and our dwellyng places cleane and pleasant, voide of corruption or infection, as by gods grace I will truly make my medicinies that I haue written" (55). Once again, the intersection between medicine and theology is evident as the apothecary wishes God to correct sanitation following medical guidelines so as to avoid plague infection. But the conversation between Crispine and Medicus also demonstrates a separation between the medical and theological worlds. While discussing Antonius's prognosis, Crispine asks, "Lorde, how this gentleman hath loued you well in his life; if he dooe depart this present worlde, will ye not be present at his buriall, Maister doctour?" (55). Medicus responds, "He loued me as I loued hym, He me for healthe, and I hym for money; And thei which are preseruers of the life of manne, ought not to be present at the death or buriall of the same man, therefore I haue taken my leaue, I warrente you Crispine; I will retourne to hym no more"(55–56). Medicus sees his role in relationship to the active life and serves only those who are living. The doctor is of little service to those that are dead or about to die.

Bullein demonstrates that a certain amount of watered-down medical knowledge, particularly about health regimens, is necessary for the common person when he returns the reader to Civis and Uxor who have departed from the city and are attempting to rejoin their children. Civis says,

> I heare a doctour of Phisicke saie that one called Galen, in a booke of Triacle, to one Pison, his friend, that the Pestilence was like a monsterous hungrie beast, deuouryng and eatyng not a fewe, but sometymes whole cities that by resperation or drawyng in their breath do take the poisoned aire. He lauded Hypocrates, whiche saieth that to remoue from the infected ayre into a cleaner, thereby, saieth he, thei did not draw in more foule ayre, and this was his onely remedie for the plague: to them that did remaine he commaunded not onelie simple wood to be burned within the Citie of Athens, but also most sweete flowers and spices, perfumes, as gummes and ointments, to purge the ayre. (57)

Civis reiterates common Galenic claims concerning the cleanness of the air and the benefits of pleasant smells. He defends his decision to flee the city by citing numerous biblical stories where the characters fled and God rewarded them (57). The connection between the medical information and biblical justification is that God's meaning for the plague is difficult to interpret. Through God's will, He provides medical knowledge about how to protect oneself from the plague. He also protects certain people in biblical stories by having them flee the city He is punishing. The essential question Civis is dealing with is the problem of interpretation. Is he supposed to use the medical information on the transmission of plague and the textual evidence on the benefits of flight to save his body or will the use of that information demonstrate that he loves life too much and therefore damns his soul?

Civis chooses a physical, rather than spiritual solution to the presence of plague. He packs up his family and his servant Roger. The conversation between Civis and Roger demonstrates the connection between illness, emotion and the divine reason for plague. Roger tells a tale about a fox, and stops from telling Civis the epitaph or the dead person's name because "you will be angrie then" (71). Civis responds, "Surely I will giue no place to anger to chafe my blod; it is perilous in the pestilent time. For next to seruyng of Almighte God, and my Christian dutie to my neighbour, I will geue my self onely to mirthe, which is the greatest iewll of this world" (71). According to Civis, anger mixes the blood up and lends the body to sickness. Doctors, as we have seen, often prescribed tales of mirth and pleasant thoughts and experiences as ways to keep the body healthy. The connection between emotion and health is not that the wrong emotion from the outside will come and harm the body. For the people of the sixteenth century, the predilection toward certain diseases is inherent. In other words, by becoming angry, a person may stir up his blood and irritate his body so that his humoral balance is changed, thereby bringing on a disease. The physical humor is not the problem; it is the emotions that cause that humor to become present. In other words, it is the spirituality of the person that influences the humoral balance and, in turn, the health of the individual. Our modern medical community subscribes to a belief that by weakening our immune system, we allow more opportunity for germs to invade an otherwise healthy organism. This is a markedly different way to view disease. For the sixteenth-century people, disease is inside; it is something the body has an inborn predisposition to.

In Early Modern medicine, disease remains clearly connected to sin. Roger continues by telling Civis what type of person the plague is punishing. Roger says that plague is caused by "[T]hat vile trade of Vsurie, procuryng Gods vengeaunce in castyng the pestilence vpon cities, tounes, and countries; causing pouertie, breakyng vp houses most aunciente, sellyng to lende vpon gaine destroying hospitalie with infinite incombraunces, by forfiture, statutes, &c" (71–72). In this passage, Roger says usury has brought about the plague. Roger is also the person most enamored with the idea that this plague demonstrates the end of the world. Throughout his long discussion with Civis, he tells of many monsters and strange signs that represent the end of the world: "I think the daie of Dome is at hande. Euery man in a maner is fallen into loue with hymselfe, either of his proper persone or apparell" (78). Roger explains that humans have lost their humanity and that plague is here to correct man's sins. Roger seems to demonstrate an older idea of plague. He believes that plague is a sign of the Apocalypse, and many of his actions throughout the dialogue are humorous, lending to the idea that his ideas should not be taken seriously because they are out of date.

Civis most demonstrates the change in interpretation of the plague from the Middle Ages to the Renaissance, for he finds out that the plague does not represent the end of the world. Instead, plague is a natural event controlled by God. Both Roger and Civis see Death approaching them (113). Uxor reminds her husband, "[R]emember I am yonge, and with childe; also you are well stricken in yeres. Therefore plaie the man, and take Roger with you, and intreate him; giue hym an hundreth poundes, and if hee will needes haue you, yet for Goddes sake be not acknowen that I am here, for fear that he kill me and your childe also" (114–15). Civis realizes that he cannot outrun death any longer and submits to him. Mors speaks,

> You are well overtaken, I am glad that wee are mette together; I haue seen you since you were borne; I haue threatened you in all your sicknesse, but you did neuer see me nor remembred me before this daie; neither had I power to haue taken you with me vntill nowe. For I haue Commission to strike you with this blacke dart, called the pestilence; my maister hath so commaunded me. (115)

Civis begs to pay his debts before dying and Mors says, "I must dipatche, and strike you with this blacke Darte; I haue muche businesse to doe with the other twoo Dartes" (116). Civis asks what the other two darts are, and Mors replies that they are famine and war (116). Mors continues by saying that no human is more powerful than he is: "be thei neuer so noble, riche, strong, wise, learned, or counnyng in Physicke, thei shall neuer preuaile against me, but I will ouercome theim" (117).

Finally, Civis asks, "What is the cause, O fearful death, that thou dooest scourge the face of the yearth with thy dartes, and who hath sente thee for that purpose?" (117). Mors replies that both the Philosopher and the Poet are mistaken and that he comes "by chaunce to mortall things" or "through the concourse of the starres" (117). Instead, he is

> the messanger of God, his scourge and crosse to all fleshe, good and badde, and am the ende of life, which doe separate the bodie from the soule. I am no feigned thyng by the wise braines of the Philosophers; but onelie through the disobedience of your firste Parentes, Adam and Eua, through whose fault all fleshe is corupted and subjecte to mee Death; for through synne came Death. (118)

Death, and therefore Pestilence, according to Mors, is simply an unexceptional part of the life cycle. This is an important difference from the literary authors who saw bubonic plague as one of the signs of Revelations. For Bullein, pestilence is not a unique event. Civis underscores this sentiment: "But now doe I see who so escapeth honger and the sworde, shal be ouertaken with the pestilence" (119). In other words, if Mors does not get the individual one way, he will get him another.

This is not to say that pestilence was no longer viewed as a sign of God's anger at man's sins. Civis sends Roger for the theologian in order to perform Last Rites. Roger goes and gets the theologian but leaves saying, "I will not return to my master againe, he will dye on this Plague. My Dame will haue newe Wedlocke within sixe weekes, and as the worlde goeth now adaies, she will think it long; out of sight out of mynde" (122). This passage demonstrates that Bullein's vision is not apocalyptic, because life continues after Civis's death. When Theologus arrives at Civis's deathbed, Civis asks him what is the cause of sin. It would appear that Civis has confused Mors's lecture on sin and ascribed the cause of sin to God. Theologus corrects him by saying, "The deuill was the first cause of synne" and "God is not the aucthour or cause of synne, for he did so much abhorre the same, that nothing could pacifie his wrathe under Heauen, no merite or woorke, but onelie the bloudde of Jesus Christe his Soone" (124–5). Civis is now clear that God did not create sin or authorize it. Sin, according to Theologus, is caused by the Devil and man. Theologus then begins a sermon in which he links sin and disease to God's divine plan: "Let vs repent, therefore, and tourne vnto God, that he may forgiue vs, that our synnes mai bee dooen awaie, that we maie saie, From Plague, Pestilence, and Famine, from battaile and murther, and from sodaine death, Oh Lorde, deliuer us" (134). Theologus connects pestilence to other forms of death, such as murder and sudden death, which implies that pestilence is no longer seen as the forebearer of the end of the world.

Both Lydgate and Bullein demonstrate the changing interpretation of plague in the fifteenth and sixteenth centuries. Practical and rational methods by which to analyze and protect people from disease replaced the interpretation that plague was the coming of the end of the world. The shift from apocalyptic vision to practical realism demonstrates a common human desire when faced with epidemic diseases. Humans tend to interpret all epidemics initially in light of the apocalypse. They attempt to interpret the reasons for the disease's appearance and identify the group the disease is consciously targeting. Eventually, these theories begin to lose their validity in two ways. First, others outside the "target group" are also infected, leading thus to either a new theory that the disease is not just focused on one group or that the disease is not intelligent enough to only punish the correct group.

The second way an apocalyptic vision loses its theoretical weight is when people realize that there are survivors from the epidemic. This realization allows people to recognize that the end of the world has not arrived, and that they need to deal with the disease in a practical, rational manner. Because AIDS did not kill people as quickly as plague, fewer people interpreted this disease as part of the apocalypse. Further, since the disease at first appeared to attack a marginal group, namely homosexuals and intravenous drug users, there was less panic in the community. The general belief remained that this disease was isolating and killing the guilty. Once people moved theoretically from an apocalyptic vision of the epidemic to a rational, pragmatic response, the disease moved from the unexplainable other to a normal part of human experience. In other words, the divine mystique has been taken away from the disease, and people begin to realize that one can take precautions and treatments either to avoid or recover from infection. In this light, medical authorities can advocate dietary regimens and changes in environment that can help to prevent infection. Furthermore, doctors can begin to work on prescriptions that combat the disease in those already infected.

The literary work, both poetry and prose, helps to disseminate the information from the medical authorities to lay people. Lydgate's and Bullein's works rely on contemporary medical beliefs about the six non-naturals and include both dietary modifications and ventilation concerns. Evidently people were interested in this practical information because, considering the number of manuscripts that have survived, both these works were highly popular in their time periods. Not only did the authors provide practical medical information, but they also produced it in a way that is both memorable and enjoyable. The role of literature as an effective and truthful means of communication was not under as much question in the fifteenth and sixteenth century as it is today. Literary authors of the Early Modern Period constructed a plague discourse that disseminated information to the masses in the hopes that more people would learn how to protect themselves against further infection.

Bubonic plague helped bring about a change in human response to disease. The interpretation of plague is a movement from allowing God to have total control over the disease to more of a human involvement. Even though cases of leprosy decreased in the later Middle Ages, authors continued to use the disease as a means of characterization. In the next chapter, I trace the literary uses of leprosy as a means of characterization in the Renaissance. While many of the connections between leprosy and falsification remain the same, some authors begin to confuse leprosy with syphilis, the new plague of the Renaissance. It is through this confusion that leprosy seems to be most closely linked to the sins of sexuality and lechery. Therefore, during the Renaissance one can begin to see the death of the medieval idea that leprosy represents falsifiers who threaten the community and the birth of the idea that leprosy, like syphilis, is a sexually transmitted disease that identifies those guilty of lechery. Lechery, one of the carnal sins, is under human control much more than spiritual sins. Consequently, when syphilis was interpreted as a disease punishing lechery, people also extended the interpretation to include leprosy, because both are skin diseases. This interpretation reflects a desire to take the control of disease out of the hand of God and place it in the hands of man.

CHAPTER SIX

Leprosy and Syphilis in Early Modern Literature

Bubonic plague changed how humans approached epidemic disease. Prior to the plague, Europeans conceived of disease, especially leprosy, as a divine punishment sent by God. The sins people believed God to be most angry with were spiritual sins. When the plague first struck, people applied the same interpretations to this new disease and, therefore thought the end of the world was coming unless people would repent their spiritual sins. However, when plague did not end the world, people began to approach the disease practically and pragmatically, paying particular attention to methods of protection and to prescriptions for healing. This approach took the control of the disease out of God's hands and placed it, however tenuously, in man's hands. When syphilis struck, people applied the same beliefs that prior people applied to leprosy, namely giving control of the disease to God and focusing on the spiritual sins as cause of the epidemic. Eventually, people interpreted syphilis as caused less by spiritual than carnal sins, owing primarily to the disease's eruption on the sexual organs. By moving from a spiritual-sin interpretation to a carnal-sin interpretation, one takes the power out of God's hand and places it more fully in man's hands for man's actions become the direct means of transmission. More interesting is the idea that leprosy was also brought over with syphilis and reinterpreted as a venereal disease, a movement that gives man more control over the means of transmission of that disease, too.

Two different moral meanings for leprosy exist in the sixteenth and seventeenth centuries. One follows the medieval association which links leprosy with spiritual sins that damage the social structure. The other moral track develops in relation to the new disease syphilis and connects both leprosy and syphilis to lechery, thus implying a venereal connection for both diseases. In this section, I begin by tracing works that follow the medieval idea that leprosy signifies sins that threaten the community. These works include Girolamo Fracastoro's *Syphilis*, Edmund Spenser's *The Fairie Queene*, and Francis Bacon's *Advancement of Learning*. I then demonstrate how other literary authors connect leprosy to syphilis and reconfigure leprosy's moral meaning to focus on sins of sexuality. In this second section, I examine the literary use of syphilis and leprosy in William Shakespeare's *Timon of Athens*, *2 Henry VI*, *Anthony and Cleopatra*, and *Henry V*; Ben Jonson's *Volpone*; and John Ford's *'Tis Pity She's a Whore*.

Medieval Leprosy and Its Influence on Syphilis: Fracastoro, Bacon, and Spenser

Girolamo Fracastoro was not an English author, but in any work that explores the social construction of disease, he must be included. His epic poem, *Syphilis* (1530), both provided the name of the disease and set the question of the disease's origin and means of transmission. Fracastoro's poem "is perhaps the most famous Renaissance Latin poem" and has "over one hundred editions . . . with translations into at least six languages" (Eatough 1). It also shaped the way Early Modern doctors, poets, and laypersons interpreted the new disease.

Syphilis is divided into three books. The first book examines the origin of the new disease, whether it has always existed or whether it came aboard ships from the New World. Fracastoro concludes:

> Quam tamen (aeternum quoniam dilabitur aevum)
> Non semel in terris visam, sed saepe fuisse,
> Ducendum est, quamquam nobis nec nomine nota
> Hacetenus illa fuit: quoniam longaeva vetustas
> Cuncta situ involvens, et res, et nomina delet:
> Nec monumenta patrum seri videre nepotes. (103–08)

> Yet, since the gliding stream of time is eternal, we must conclude that this plague has been seen on earth, not once but often, although up to now it has not been known to us even by name: since age with its length of years shrouds everything in decay, it destroys both objects and their names: late descendants do not see even the memorials of their forefathers. (trans. Eatough 43)

Like many of his modern historical counterparts, Fracastoro finds it difficult to see syphilis as a new disease; instead he chooses to say that this is an old disease simply forgotten by temporal human beings. Nevertheless, Fracastoro declares that across the ocean a "misera ... gens" ("unfortunate people") lives where "nullisque locis non cognita vulgo est" ("no one nor any place is known by the people" 110–11). The people of the Americas live with syphilis as a common disease; therefore, the disease is both ancient and new: ancient because it existed from the dawn of time, but new because Early Modern people forgot it.

In his second book, Fracastoro lists methods of treatment that were common to medical doctors of the sixteenth century. To avoid syphilis, people are to employ the six non-naturals listed by Galen: air, exercise and rest, sleep and waking, food and drink, repletion and excretion, and the passions.[1] Fracastoro's work makes the treatments for syphilitics authoritative. One of the most common cures was believed to be quicksilver, which Fracastoro declares helps "omnia vivo" ("all to live" II. 270). The other cure common to syphilis treatment was sweating. While Fracastoro declares that sweating works, he admits that this is a painful and humiliating treatment:

> Hic igitur totum oblinere, atque obducere corpus
> Ne obscoenum, ne turpe puta: per talia morbus
> Tollitur, et nihil esse potest obscoenius ipso.
> Parce tamen capiti, et praecordia mollia vita.
> Tum super et vittas astringe, et stuppea necte
> Vellera: dein stratis tegmento imponere multo,
> Dum sudes, foedaeque fluant per corpora guttae.
> Haec tibi bis quinis satis est iterasse diebus.
> Durum erit: at quicquid tulerit res ipsa, ferendum est.
> Aude animus. Tibi certa salus stans limine in ipso
> Signa dabit: liquefacta mali excrementa videbis
> Assidue sputo immundo fluitare per ora,
> Et largum ante pedes tabi mirabere flumen. (436–49)

> Don't consider it repulsive nor disgusting to smear and cover the whole body; by such means the disease is removed, and nothing could be more repulsive than it. Yet spare the head and avoid the soft parts before the heart. Then on top bind bandages tightly and fasten dressings made of tow; next put yourself in bed with many blankets, until you sweat and the filthy drops flow over your body. It will be enough for you to have repeated this for ten days. It will be hard: but whatever the treatment brings must be borne. Be bold in spirit. Salvation as she stands right on the threshold will give you sure signs: you will constantly see the filthy liquified excretions of the disease pouring from your lips in the dirty spittle and you will be amazed at the large streams of corrupt matter before your feet. (trans. Eatough 83–85)

As is clear from his use of value-laden words, Fracastoro believes that syphilis is a punishment connected to sin. He reads the disease as "obscoenum," "dirty or filthy"; "foedae," "shameful"; and "immundo," "filthy or foul." Moreover, the cure of the disease is seen as "salus," "health," "deliverance." Fracastoro sees the cure for this disease along lines also associated with penance. The fluids that the regimen brings forth are the corrupt and sinful matter caused by the disease. The body reflects the state of the soul, and the body must pay for its transgressions against the soul.

Syphilis's relationship with sin is firmly established in Fracastoro's work. In Book III, the poem's persona describes how the sailors to the New World became infected with syphilis. In a sacred forest in the New World, Spanish sailors decided to take target practice on the birds of the forest. A female voice speaks to the men telling them that they have sinned and that they will be subjugated to a "longa populos in libertate quietos" (III. 180). The sailors will have to endure "trials by sea and land" (III. 182).[2] After listing numerous trials, the voice finally states, "That day, when your bodies are corrupted with an ugly, unknown sickness / you will ask for help from this forest for your wretchedness / while you repent this wicked deed" (III. 190–92, my translation).[3] The sailors and their homeland are punished because they abused the sacred forests by taking the lives of the birds for pleasure. The sailors attempt to pay retribution and tribute to the gods of the Americas, but the "gens Europea" are amazed at the contagion that infected Europe (III. 248–49).

The Spanish leader then asks the native King about the disease. The King explains that his race came from the noble Atlas and that "luxury and arrogance"[4] destroyed the tribe (III. 271). God punished the people through earthquakes, famine, and pestilence. The pestilence, which few avoided, was sent down because of "Divum offensis, et Apollinis ira" and still rages in their cities (III. 284). The King continues by explaining that the person to first bring the disease was Syphilis, a shepherd, who after growing tired of the oppressive heat of one summer solstice declared to the Sun:

> Nam quid, Sol te . . . rerum patremque Deumque
> Dicimus, et sacras vulgus rude ponimus aras.
> Mactatoque bove, et pingui veneramur acerra,
> Si nostri nec cura tivi est, nec regia tangunt
> Armenta? An potuis superos vos arbitrer uri
> Invidia? Mihi pascuntur oves: vix est tibi Taurus
> Unus, vix Aries coelo (si vera feruntur)
> Unus, et armenti custos Canis arida tanti.
> Demens quin potius Regi divina facesso?
> Cui tot agri, tot sunt populi, cui lata ministrant
> Aequora, et est superis, ac Sole potentia major?
> Ille dabit facilesque auras, frigusque virentum
> Dulce feret nemorum armentis, aestumque levabit. (III. 296–309)

> Why, Sun, do we call you Father and God of all things and why do we, the ignorant masses, lay out sacred altars and worship you with sacrifice of ox and casket rich in incense, if you have no concern for us and the king's flocks do not touch your heart? Or rather am I to think that you Gods are scorched with envy? By me a thousand cattle, white as snow, are pastured, by me and a thousand sheep; you have in heaven, if reports are true, merely one Bull, one Ram—and one dried-up Bitch to guard this enormous herd.

> What a fool I am, that I don't rather perform divine rites for the king, who has so many estates, so many subjects, whom the broad seas supply and whose power is greater than the Gods and the Sun. The king will grant favouring breezes, he will bring sweet coolness of green groves to our herds and lighten the burden of the heat. (Eatough 101)

Syphilis then makes altars to King Alcithous and praises him as a god. Because of Syphilis's actions, God infects the air that in turn affects Syphilis and gives him disfiguring sores (III. 324–28). The plague continues to infect the city and the people, even killing the King in the story (III. 323–24). Finally, the native people ask Ammerice, a nymph of the forest, how to cure the disease. She states,

> Spreti vos O, vos numina Solis Exercent: nulli fas est se aequare Deorum
> Mortalem: date thura Deo, et sua ducite sacra,
> Et numen placate, iras non proferet ultra.
> Quam tulit, aeterna est, nec jam revocabilis unquam
> Pestis erit: quincunque solo nascetur in isto,
> Sentiet, ille lacus Sygios, fatumque severum
> Juravit. Sed enim, si jam medicamina certa
> Expetitis, niveam magnae mactate juvencam
> Junoni, magnae nigrantem occcidite vaccam
> Telluri: illa dabit foelicia semina ab alto:
> Haec viridem educet foelici semina ab alto:
> Haec viridem educet foelicia semina sylvam:
> Unde salus (III. 339–51)

> You, oh, you are being tried by the power of the Sun you despised; with none of the Gods is it right for a moral to equate himself: give incense to God, and conduct the rites which are his, and appease his power, then he will not carry his anger further. But the plague which he has brought on is eternal and can never now be revoked. Whoever is born on that soil will feel it; God has sworn this by the Stygian lakes and stern fate. But if now you desire a sure treatment, offer a white heifer to mighty Juno, slaughter a black cow to the mighty Earth: Juno will give seeds of happiness from on high; the Earth will train up a green wood from the happy seed: whence your salvation. (trans. Eatough 103)

The seed that Juno gives is from the Guaiacum tree, a tree that was believed by both sixteenth-century doctors and laypersons to cure syphilis. When the King finishes the story, the infected Spanish offer tribute to the Sun and take Guaiacum trees back to Europe with them to cure those infected. Fracastoro ends his poem by praising the tree and hoping that it will cure the disease. Unlike his assurances for quicksilver and sweating, there is no assurance that Guaiacum is a cure all; there is only a hope that it is.

The connection Fracastoro makes between syphilis and sin is markedly the same as that between leprosy and sin in the Bible. Like Uzziah in the Old Testament, who attempts to offer incense to God as a priest would, Syphilis in Fracastoro's poem does not seem to realize that he should praise God rather than man. God becomes angry at man's lack of respect and punishes the community of men. Fracastoro creates a man, Syphilis, who does not know his social place and who is guilty of blasphemy. More importantly, the entire community is in need of correction, and unlike leprosy, the disease affects all the people. Once unleashed, God can no longer take it away, but he does provide medicines that will relieve the suffering. Most important in Fracastoro's work is that syphilis is connected to sins that affect the community, such as pride, envy and blasphemy, spiritual sins commonly associated with leprosy. As Hays writes, "'Syphilis' was a shepherd who brought the pox on himself by his acts of blasphemy, illustrating that the connection of the pox with sex was still not universally accepted" (67).

The medieval idea that leprosy was a punishment for sins that threaten the community remains evident in literature of the sixteenth and seventeenth centuries. *The Faerie Queene* (1596), Spenser's romantic epic, employs many structures common to literature of the Middle Ages. The moral nature of Spenser's work is evident in the allegorical association of the knights of the first three books: Holiness, Temperance and Chastity. But Spenser's work need not be taken on a purely allegorical level. Especially in Book I of *The Faerie Queene*, Spenser delights the reader with a wonderful description of Duessa's House of Pride and the sicknesses that accompany certain sins. While it is possible to read these diseases metaphorically, it is also possible to read them literally because the authoritative medical tradition stated that specific diseases, such as leprosy, were caused by specific sins. Throughout Book I, Spenser portrays the dangers of allowing one's perceptions to govern one's choices. While these perceptions may appear to be accurate, they may inherently lead the person to further sin. Disease, for Spenser, also functions along similar lines because a person may have the disease internally without displaying external signs. Consequently, the person could continue to infect others while portraying himself or herself as healthy and free of sin.

In Book I, Canto 4, Redcrosse knight is led to the House of Pride from whence few have escaped:

> Great troupes of people traveild thitherward
> Both day and night, of each degree and place,
> But few returnèd, having scapèd hard,
> With balefull beggerie, or foule disgrace,
> Which euer after in most wretched case,
> Like loathsome lazars, by the hedges lay. (3.1–6)

Those who attempt to leave the House of Pride can do so, but they will be punished by either poverty or disgrace. Through a simile, Spenser connects both poverty and disgrace to the lepers that lay around the House of Pride. It is a logical choice for what Spencer wants to describe. The leper needs to beg from the general public because by social edict he or she is now a marginal figure outside the community. Also, lepers represent some form of social disgrace; they are the social outcasts.

Even though Spencer was writing well after both the outbreak of syphilis and the apparent semantic integration of leprosy and syphilis, he maintains common medieval connections between leprosy and sin. After the Redcrosse knight enters the House of Pride with Duessa, Lucifera is the first person described in this horrible pageant of the seven deadly sins. That Lucifera is the epitome of Pride is demonstrated both by her attire and by the allusion to peacocks in her pageant "that excell in pride" (I.iv.17.8).[5] Regarding this image, Samuel Chew states, "Spenser does not assign to Pride the peacock which is often this Sin's emblem, but in likening her coach to 'Junoes golden chaire ... drawne of faire Pecocks,' he implies this association" (42). The prideful Duessa is the first to be described but actually ends the pageant (Chew 46). After the narrator describes the prideful Lucifera, he begins to describe the first member of the pageant: "sluggish Idlenesse the nourse of sin" (I.iv.18.6). The narrator then describes each sin and the disease that sin begets. Gluttony comes next and suffers from dropsy (I.iv.21–23) and next to him rides Lechery. Lechery suffers not from leprosy, but from syphilis:

> Which lewdnesse fild him with reprochfull paine
> Of that fowle evil, which all men reprove,
> That rots the marrow, and consumes the braine:
> Such one was Lecherie, the third of all the traine. (I.iv.26.6–9)

Lechery is the third person in Pride's pageant, and he clearly suffers from syphilis characterized by the reference to a disease that affects the bones and brains of the victims.

Spenser's order of the Seven Deadly Sins also follows medieval traditions. In *The Seven Deadly Sins*, Bloomfield argues that Spenser's pageant's "general scheme is, of course, medieval, and the most notable of Spenser's English forebearers is Gower" (241). Spenser is relying on the traditional Gregorian method of presenting the Seven Deadly Sins, a method Gower also employed in *Mirrour de l'Omme*.[6] In *Mirrour de l'Omme*, Gower presents the sins in the following order: Pride, Envy, Anger, Sloth, Avarice, Gluttony, and Lechery.[7] This rendering for the most part is Gregory the Great's (d.604 A.D.), and can be divided up into two categories: spiritual and carnal. Spenser's work is surely medieval, in this sense, for he orders his sins according to medieval custom and he connects leprosy to envy, not lechery.

Spenser's pageant can be divided into three categories; Gower's version cannot. Spenser follows a similar Gregorian pattern, but Spenser's order is inverted because Pride, while described first by the narrator, ends the pageant. Spenser's order is Sloth, Gluttony, Lechery, Avarice, Envy, Wrath, and Pride, and falls into an easily identifiable order. Sloth, Gluttony, and Lechery are the carnal sins, the sins of the flesh. Avarice is the sin of the world, and Envy, Wrath, and Pride are sins of the Devil (Chew 46). One need only recall Dante's *Divine Comedy* to demonstrate the hierarchy of the seven deadly sins. Sins of the body, like Lechery and Gluttony, are placed in the second and third pouches of Hell, respectively. These pouches are right next to Limbo, the first pouch of Hell, and many pouches away from the worse sins, such as Pride.[8] Similarly, in *The Castle of Perseverance*, a fifteenth-century morality play, the playwright classifies the sins into those of the Devil (pride, envy, and wrath), Flesh (gluttony, lechery, sloth), and World (avarice). It would appear that Spenser is truer to the order of the *Castle* than Gower, at least as far as the organization of the sins under collective headings. More importantly, Spenser relies on medieval sensibility for his organization and characterization of the Seven Deadly Sins, and this is most evident in how he describes the sin of envy.

In relation to sins of the word, Spenser demonstrates the medieval idea that leprosy was a punishment for sins of language that threatened the community, rather than sins of the body. Near the end of the parade of sins in the House of Pride comes "malicious Envie" (262). The narrator summarizes that Envy:

> ... hated all good workes and vertuous deeds,
> And him no lesse, that nay like did use,
> And who with gracious bread the hungry feeds,
> His almes for want of faith he doth accuse;
> So every good to bad he doth abuse:
> And eke the verse of famous Poets witt
> He does backebite, and spitefull poison spues
> From leprous mouth on all, that ever writt:
> Such one vile Envie was, that fifte in row did sitt. (I.iv.32.1–9)

Spenser is drawing on a tradition in which leprosy represents the sin of Envy, a sin that threatens the stability of the community. Further, Spenser plays on the common cultural mythology that leprosy could be passed from person to person through infected air. Spenser draws the reader's attention to the idea that the words Envy spews, words that backbite and are spiteful, have the potential to infect everyone just as leprosy was believed to be transmitted from a leper to a healthy person through the air. As Chew writes, "Elsewhere in *The Faerie Queene*, Spenser assigns some of Envy's traits to Slander; the Sin has, indeed, a close affiliation with Slander, Detraction, Calumny, and Deceit, as is apparent in the various "Calumny of Apelles" painting" (52). Inappropriate language, therefore, threatens the stability of the community, as does leprosy that threatens the health of the body.

Francis Bacon also employs the connection between leprosy and language and the ability of both to threaten the community. Bacon's discussion of leprosy brings these ideas out of the poetic realm and into that of philosophy and science. His text further demonstrates that the fear of lepers was part of the social fabric, not simply a poetic device. In Book I of *Advancement of Learning* (1605), Bacon describes the limitations of human learning and the common distempers that prevent further learning. When discussing theology, Bacon argues that many of the laws of Moses have both a natural and moral rationale. Evidently, Bacon sees the works of the Bible as having both scientific and social value. He believes that the works of Leviticus identify leprosy because it is contagious and a reflection of an individual's moral status. Therefore, one can see how deeply ingrained into the collective consciousness was the idea that diseases reflect sins. The disease becomes the social text by which others are warned of possible danger. As evidence, Bacon uses

> the law of the leprosy where it is said, "If the whiteness have overspread the flesh, the patient may pass abroad for clean; but if there be any whole flesh remaining, he is to be shut up for unclean"; one of them noteth a principle of nature, that putrefaction is more contagious before maturity than after: another noteth a position of moral philosophy, that men abandoned to vice do not so much corrupt manners, as those that are half good and half evil. (I. 9)

Bacon demonstrates some important ideas about the construction and knowledge of diseases. He declares that those who are recently infected are the most dangerous on both moral and physical levels. In relation to moral issues, those who are not fully embraced by their disease are the most dangerous because it may be possible to hide the signs of the disease and thereby pass as morally pure. In Sontag's terminology, these people would have passports to both the kingdom of the healthy and ill. Human beings tend to be most uncomfortable with this kind of social interpretation of illness. However, if disease has taken over the entire body, everyone can read the body as text and know that this person is not to be trusted. Chaucer's Summoner exemplifies Bacon's belief about disease that has not fully erupted. The Summoner's disease is barely noticeable which makes him more of a threat to the community than a person with confirmed leprosy. The Summoner's involvement with the children of the community furthers those social fears.

Bacon's text also demonstrates an important idea in the scientific framework of disease. As Bacon states, most contagious are those infected but whose disease has not reached maturity. Bacon states that individuals whose disease has matured or those whose disease has appeared and apparently gone away are not contagious. The Early Modern concept of potential disease transmission influenced how many people became infected because those with full-blown illnesses were deemed not to be contagious. Furthermore, this form of disease recognition demonstrates how strongly this culture relied on the body as text. People whose bodies were free from visual symptoms were considered healthy. Other people whose disease was evident on the skin were easy to identify and, therefore, the healthy could protect themselves against the ill. The ones whose disease had not yet appeared on the body were the greatest threat to the community for they could pass as healthy and thereby infect those who were unaware.

It would appear that on the evidence of Spenser and Bacon, a line of thought that connected lepers with envy and slander continued through the sixteenth and seventeenth centuries. But leprosy is also connected to syphilis in this period, and while it is difficult to locate a single literary work or time period when leprosy was firmly connected to sins of sexuality, it is possible to observe a development of the association over time. I have already demonstrated how Fracastoro constructed syphilis along similar lines to that leprosy, especially syphilis's link to blasphemy. In the next part of this chapter, I examine how the discourse surrounding leprosy and syphilis becomes conflated, and how leprosy comes to be interpreted primarily as caused by lechery.

JONSON, SHAKESPEARE, AND FORD

By the sixteenth and seventeenth centuries, authors increasingly associated syphilis to the sins of sexuality. Leprosy remained in a problematic area where authors sometimes connected it to sins of the community and other times connected it to sins of sexuality. Ben Jonson's *Volpone* (1606) demonstrates both the role of syphilis as a representation of sinful sexuality and the belief that leprosy reflects sins of the community. The connection between syphilis and sin is clearly established in Act 1 of *Volpone* when Mosca demonstrates Volpone's unconscious state to Corvino. In Volpone's ear, Mosca shouts, "The pox approach, and add to your diseases, / If it would send you hence the sooner, sir, / For your incontinence, it hath deserved it" (I.5 52–4). The connection between sin and disease is evident. Mosca declares that it would be logical for Volpone to suffer from syphilis because of his incontinence. More importantly, according to the *Oxford English Dictionary*, Jonson is the first poet to use "incontinence" to refer to an unchaste person in *Every Man in His Humour* (1598): "O, old, incontinent, dost thou not shame / When all thy powers in chastity are spent / To have a mind so hot?" (4.8). Being incontinent points to the development of the idea that syphilis is a venereal disease, because incontinent people would not be true to one lover, but would have many.

The idea that syphilis is a venereal disease is underscored in Act II when Nano, a dwarf, sings a song to Volpone, who has disguised himself as a mountebank doctor called Scoto Mantuano pushing a cure-all. The song is a pitch to other people to buy the tonic that cures everything. Nano sings, "Would you live free from all diseases? / Do the act your mistress pleases, / Yet fright all aches from your bones?" (II.2 214–6). Aching bones is a common symptom of syphilis and often authors refer to the disease as bone ache. The connection between syphilis and sexuality is unmistakable: If people buy this tonic, though, they can have sex and remain immune to syphilis.[9]

A connection between disease and sin is furthered in this play when Corvino states that no medication can work unless the person creating the medication is pure. Voltore and Corbaccio return with the elixir, and Mosca tells Corvino, a local merchant, about how it brought Volpone back to life. Corvino questions the power of this drug because "... I / Known him a common rogue, come fiddling in / To the osteria with a tumbling whore" (II.6 12–14). Corvino is defaming the mountebank doctor, Scoto Mantuano, whom Volpone played when attempting to pawn the elixir. Corvino knows each ingredient and its effects. The value of the medicine is clearly degraded by the actions of the curer. In other words, Corvino does not believe Mosca because Scoto is lecherous.

As diseases become endemic, terminology also develops and changes. Mosca explains how the medication was applied: "they poured into his ears / Some in his nostriles, and recovered him; / Applying but the fricace" (II.6 21–3). Corvino replies, "Pox o' that fricace!"(II.6 24). This use of "pox" as a curse demonstrates that syphilis was integrated into Early Modern vocabulary according to its metaphorical associations. By Jonson's time syphilis had become such a common part of life that it was used metaphorically.

Other diseases are also used as curses, but not in the same way as pox was in the sixteenth and seventeenth centuries. Leprosy is used as a curse when Volpone tries to seduce and rape Celia, Corvino's wife. After reciting to her a love poem and arguing the benefits to her of an adulterous affair, Celia pleads that Volpone should either let her escape or kill her. If he will do neither of these actions, then she asks:

> If you will deign me neither of these graces,
> Yet feed your wrath, sir, rather than your lust
> (It is a vice comes nearer manliness)
> And punish that unhappy crime of Nature
> Which you miscall my beauty: flay my face,
> Or poison it with ointments, for seducing
> Your blood to this rebellion. Rub these hands
> With what may cause an eating leprosy
> E'en to my bones and marrow; anything
> That may disfavour me, save in my honour. (III.7 248–57)

Celia's request to ask for leprosy as a punishment demonstrates that leprosy was still connected to sins other than sex, because leprosy would punish her beauty but still allow her to retain her honor. Jonson could have had Celia beg for syphilis, a disease that would effectively destroy her beauty also. But that disease, at least in Jonson's mind, would have been linked to her honor, her sexual honor. Consequently, what one can see through her statement is that sexual honor may be more important socially for a woman than any other type of honor.

Jonson's *Volpone* also demonstrates the changing social uses of Lazar hospitals now that leprosy was not as common. In Act IV of *Volpone*, a knight named Sir Politick Would-Be offers a new way for Peregrine to quarantine ships. Quarantining began during the Middle Ages with the advent of the Black Death. Ships from countries in which plague is endemic must remain anchored for forty days. Sir Politick declares his problem:

> My next is, how to enquire, and be resolved,
> By present demonstration, whether a ship,
> Newly arrived from Syria, or from
> Any suspected part of all the Levant,
> Be guilty of the plague: and where they use
> To lie out forty, fifty days, sometimes,
> About the Lazaretto, for their trial;
> I'll save that charge and loss unto the merchant,
> And in an hour clear the doubt. (IV.1 100–8)

Although he does not want to use a Lazaretto at all for quarantine, he does suggest that Lazarettos were being used for diseases other than leprosy, in this case plague. Lazar hospitals had other purposes than holding leprous persons (Rawcliffe 14–15). Further, at least by Jonson's time, the lazar hospital became commercialized. Instead of being torn down, the hospital served the community by continuing to protect it from other diseases.

The desire to protect the society from disease had severe effects on the market and economy. The effects of quarantine on the economy pushed medical science to develop tests for disease, rather than relying on the body as the text. If someone could develop a test, which would use something other than the body to determine disease, like that of Sir Politick's onion, then the economy would improve because goods would not have to stay in holding for forty days. Jonson's play demonstrates the desire for a test for disease. Because of the pressure of capitalism, Politick offers a new way of testing for plague. By cutting onions into halves, Politick believes that the onions

> Attract the infection, and your bellows blowing
> The air upon him, will show instantly,
> By this change of colour, if there be contagion;
> Or else remain as fair as at the first.
> Now it is known, 't is nothing. (IV.1 122–6)

Politick's test can be seen as a way to replace the body as text with some other text. The main impetus for this test is monetary, because a quarantined fleet causes merchants to lose money. However, the desire to make money also produces its own disease.

The connection between money and syphilis is very important in many of Shakespeare's works. Scholars have investigated the use of disease and medicine in Shakespeare's plays more than in any other Renaissance literary author's. Three critical works explore the role of medicine in Shakespeare's plays. In *Shakespeare and Medicine* (1959), R. R. Simpson, a medical doctor, was the first to catalogue Shakespeare's references to disease, doctors, and medical thought. More recently, F. David Hoeniger, in *Medicine and Shakespeare in the English Renaissance* (1992), expands Simpson's work to examine both the literal and metaphoric references to disease and medicine. Hoeniger concludes that while Shakespeare was knowledgeable about medical ideas of his time, he was not the originator of these ideas, as Simpson implied. Rather, Shakespeare was part of a social system and passed this knowledge on through his works (Hoeniger 12–13). The knowledge that he had about disease came from a variety of authorities, including medical and theological. Part of the knowledge that Shakespeare passed on was the concept that leprosy and syphilis were similar diseases that punished people for specific sins.

Unlike Hoeniger and Simpson, who deal with the entire Shakespearean canon and all of medicine, other critics have turned to examine one disease within a few specific plays. In *Shakespeare and the New Disease: The Dramatic Function of Syphilis in Troilus and Cressida, Measure for Measure, and Timon of Athens* (1989), Greg W. Bentley examines actual references and potential allusions to syphilis in these plays. Bentley argues that each work is connected to social problems that were present in Renaissance England. According to Bentley, *Troilus and Cressida* is primarily concerned with sexual commercialism common in London during Shakespeare's time (217). *Measure for Measure* examines "the nature of justice and its proper administration, especially with regard to the distinction between personal slander and sedition" (217). Finally *Timon of Athens* "focus[es] on the personal and economic destruction caused by usury" (217). Bentley is mainly concerned with attempting to show a unity in Shakespeare's "problem plays," and he often treats disease on a metaphoric level. Bentley does a good job of providing the major critical camps of interpretation for these plays; however, he is not necessarily concerned with the way Shakespeare's uses leprosy and syphilis as part of a social construction. By using Bentley's work and by reexamining Shakespeare's text, I will demonstrate Shakespeare's ambivalence with respect to leprosy and syphilis as sexual diseases. More importantly, these references to diseases can be seen on a literal as well as metaphoric level and as part of an overall social interpretation of disease common to the sixteenth and seventeenth centuries.

The title character of *Timon of Athens* (1608) is Shakespeare's study in the evolution of a misanthrope whose Christian charity evolves into prodigal usury. Avarice is the main sin in this play, and Timon's friends are shown as opportunists whose friendship lasts only as long as they can borrow his money and use his powerful social standing. When Timon apparently runs out of money and loses his social position, his friends quickly abandon him, causing his change in attitude toward mankind. Bentley says that Shakespeare hopes that "if his work cannot immediately compel malefactors who commit the offenses he has portrayed to change their behavior, it can at least raise his audiences' level of awareness about such evil and therefore partially equip them with an intellectual defense for guarding against these vices" (145). These social vices that Shakespeare describes are also related to a variety of diseases that are sent to correct society. In Act 5, scene 1, Timon states, "What is amiss, plague and infection mend!" (220). The presence of disease in the play is not metaphoric; it is meant to be taken literally. For Early Modern people, disease represents and reflects the problems of the society, and it is the corrector of an errant society. The question is, what is the actual problem that the disease is trying to cure? In *Timon of Athens*, the problem seems to be lending practices.

One of the problems of Shakespeare's society was the growing money-lending business. However, the problems of usury extend far beyond simple lending. Poets and painters attempt to flatter Timon in order to better their social standing. By Act V, Timon has also described them as guilty of usury. Bentley states, "In fact, [poets and painters] represent the most abject kind, since they are shown to be exceptionally conscious of what they are doing" (156). Bentley further argues that usury in Shakespeare's time extends beyond false friendship and flattery into prostitution (159–60). According to Bentley, Renaissance social critics Thomas Lodge and George Whetstone saw businessmen tricking young gentlemen out of land and money by appealing to their "sexual appetites" (Bentley 159). In *The Enemie of Unthryftness*, Whetstone devotes individual discussions to both "Brokers of Bawdry" and "Brokers of Money," and ends his discussion on the "Sanctuaries of Iniquitie":

> These wicked houses first nurseth our young gentlemen in pride, and acquainteth them with sundrie shifting companions, whereof one sort consume him with lecherie, an other sort by brocadge bringeth him in debt, and out of credit, then awayteth covetousness and usurie to sease upon his living, and the uncivill Sergeant upon his libertie. To ruine is thus brought the gentleman, a great estate and strength of this Realme, principally by frequenting of dicing house. (qtd. in Bentley 159–60)

Evidently, usury by Renaissance standards was an umbrella term that covered money lending, false friendship, flattery, and prostitution. All five of these sins have the ability to threaten the society, and it is Shakespeare that links all five together in *Timon of Athens* by relating them to syphilis.

But leprosy is also evident in this play, and upon reexamination of the text, one can see that Shakespeare uses leprosy as a representation of false language. Throughout the play, Shakespeare draws on the medieval notion that leprosy represents those individuals who threaten the community through language, particularly slander. One of the references to leprosy occurs when Apemantus and Timon meet at Timon's cave and argue over their villainous natures in Act 4, Sc. 3. In this scene, Apemantus curses Timon by saying, "A plague on thee! Thou art too bad to curse" (365). Timon responds, "All villains that do stand by thee are pure" (366), to which Apemantus states, "There is no leprosy but what thou speak'st" (367). These insults are a series of contrasts in which the individual is worse than the sin. Timon declares that criminals look pure next to Apemantus, and Apemantus links leprosy to Timon's false words. In other words, lepers who are known for their false language appear to be true in relation to Timon's false words.

The language Timon uses is metaphorically leprous, which means that Apemantus is purer than Timon makes him out to be. Timon responds to Apemantus's leprosy jab by saying, "If I name thee / I'll beat thee, but I should infect my hands" (368–69). Timon demonstrates the common belief that leprosy is easily contagious. More importantly, Timon declares that what he says is not slanderous. Thus, through indirection, it is Apemantus who is making slanderous statements for he is the one who could cause leprosy in Timon through physical contact rather than verbal battle. Apemantus responds to this jibe: "I would my tongue could rot them off" (370). Bentley sees this line as representative of allusions to rabies common in Elizabethan England (181). However, this line could also refer to the idea that lepers' bodies appear to people to be rotting on the outside. The "them" Apemantus is referring to are Timon's hands. Apemantus accepts the idea that he could be given leprosy through his slander, and then he wishes that he could use his slanderous tongue to rot Timon's hands off. What is underscored is the common medieval belief that lepers are being punished for the language they use, and the tongue therefore is the weapon best able to bring about leprosy. As syphilis punishes an individual by the very means through which he or she transgressed, so too does leprosy use the implement that birthed the disease. Shakespeare believes that leprosy reflects those guilty of false language, of slander; similarly, Bacon connected leprosy to language. The disease's connection to false language demonstrates a medieval association between the leprosy and sin of the social order. However, because Timon associates false language with usury and because syphilis is associated with usury, the two diseases become closely allied. They are also linked to the sins of money and sex.

The connection between money, sex, and syphilis is most clearly stated in Act 2, scene 2, when the Fool and Apemantus discuss the state of usury. The Fool asks the Servants, "Are you three usurers' men?" (99). After the servants respond affirmatively, the Fool states, "I think no usurer but has a fool to his servant; my mistress is one, and I am her fool. When men come to borrow of your masters, they approach sadly and go away merry, but they enter my mistress's house merrily and go away sadly" (101–05). Usury functions in two ways here. For the people who come to the moneylender's house, they approach sadly needing money, but leave happily with a loan. In opposition, men looking for sex approach the mistress merrily but leave sadly because the mistress is a prostitute and, most likely, gave the man a venereal disease (Bentley 161). Usury, one recalls, is a sin associated with leprosy in the Old Testament. Here we see the expansion of usury to include prostitution and the development of an association with this sin and syphilis.

A similar connection between the sins associated with leprosy and syphilis is made in Act 4 where Timon's misanthropic attitudes are firmly established. Timon curses the free-livers with disease by saying,

> . . . Lust and liberty
> Creep in the minds and marrows of our youth,
> That 'gainst the stream of virtue that may strive
> And drown themselves in riot! Itches, blains,
> Sow all th' Athenian bosoms, and their crop
> Be general leprosy! Breath infect breath,
> That their society as their friendship, may
> Be merely poison! (4.1.25–32)

Within this passage lies the medieval social construction surrounding leprosy, a social construction that argues that the sins that threaten society can eventually bring about the end of the world. In this case, leprosy is meant to destroy the entire society through the infection of the young. Timon hopes that the sins of the youths will fester in their bosoms and come forth as a crop of leprosy that will infect the entire society. Leprosy here is connected to words, particularly to how the disease is transmitted from breath to breath. Furthermore, the disease is lodged in the person's heart, which implies the victim's true nature. Again we see the belief in a humoral system of disease in which a disease lies within a person and needs only the right set of circumstances to erupt. The right circumstances are ones that go "against the stream of virtue." Furthermore, Athenian friendship is seen as a poison, because the words of friendship are not true. Leprosy for Timon represents a disease that threatens the stability of the society, primarily through language.

Timon also connects lust to the list of possible sins associated with leprosy. As the opening of the quotation above suggests, the young men guilty of usury are interested in lust and liberty. Within this line lies the idea that usury relates to both prostitution and money. Through prostitution, young men satisfy their lust, and through flattery and coercion, young men get money in order to be financially free. When Timon states how "Lust and liberty / creep into the minds and marrow," he alludes to syphilis, which attacks the mind and the bones of the one infected. Concerning these lines, Bentley states,

> The disease that resulted from "lust and liberty," i.e., sexual license, is clearly syphilis, especially if it "creeps" into the mind and marrow of the bones. Many Renaissance medical writers point out that syphilis caused madness and corrupted the bones. Severe itching and burning, as Francisco Lopez de Villalobos says, were also common symptoms of the disease. Lastly, more than one Renaissance doctor describes how syphilis, after its initial virulent attack, supposedly degenerates into other diseases, particularly leprosy. Besides wanting Athens thrown into a general state of chaos, then, Timon wants to destroy its inhabitants completely by having each of them subjected to a painful and incurable case of syphilis. (191–92)

Moreover, Shakespeare is demonstrating the way syphilis's and leprosy's social constructions are being conflated in the late sixteenth and early seventeenth centuries. While leprosy was believed to be a divinely sent disease that protected the status quo by identifying those who threaten the community, in this case usurers, syphilis is now being associated with similar social groups. At the same time, Shakespeare is also expanding leprosy's sinful associations by connecting it to lust and lechery, while still retaining its association to false words.

Timon also uses leprosy and syphilis to demonstrate how these diseases identify problems within the society. But few people recognize the meaning of the disease and alter the behavior that the disease identifies. Consequently, Timon believes that his world is turning upside down. In Act 4 scene 3, Timon speaks about his gold:

> This yellow slave
> Will knit and break religions, blest th' accurst
> Make the hoar leprosy adored, place thieves
> And give them title, knee, and approbation
> With senators on the bench. This is it
> That makes the wappended widow wed again;
> She whom the spital house and ulcerous sores
> Would cast the gorge at, this embalms and spices
> To th' April day. Come, damnèd earth,
> Thou common whore of mankind, that puts odds
> Among the rout of nations, I will make thee
> Do thy right nature. (34–45)

Leprosy and syphilis, referred to by the spital house, are the only two diseases Timon identifies in his diatribe on the sins of money. Shakespeare also uses a homonym in an interesting play on words as he identifies characterizes leprosy as "hoar." The word identifies the color of the skin of the leper;

however, when this line would have been spoken, most people would hear the word "whore," thereby connecting the disease to sexuality rather than skin color. In this homonym lies the new meaning for leprosy. While once associated with money and sin, with the introduction of syphilis, a sexually transmitted disease, leprosy is now being associated with sex. Money makes the leper to be adored rather than scorned. And money makes the ugly, menopausal widow, with whom syphilitics from the spittle houses would be sick to be involved, voluptuous as a maiden in spring. Money, according to Timon, has turned the world upside down by making that which is dishonorable honorable. Therefore, he buries the gold deep in the earth, perhaps in ironic reference to the parable of the vineyard. Usury, sex, leprosy, and syphilis are intertwined. Both diseases are being used hyperbolically to describe how far the community strayed from the morally correct path.

Other plays by Shakespeare also swap and conflate the moral associations of syphilis and leprosy. Leprosy demonstrates false words in *2 Henry VI* (1590), especially as a disease related to social order. Humphrey, Duke of Gloucester, is the fair-minded counsel to King Henry, but Queen Margaret resents this relationship between Gloucester and the King. Margaret and Suffolk both represent royalty that cares little for justice and that oppresses the masses. After Suffolk designs the murder of Gloucester, the King mourns the death of his best adviser. In Act 3 scene 2, Queen Margaret responds to the King's concern for Gloucester by saying, "Be woe for me, more wretched than he is. / What, dost thou turn away and hide thy face? / I am no loathsome leper. Look on me" (3.2 73–5). There are many possible readings of these lines. On a literal level, Margaret is saying that she should be the King's comfort, as Gloucester had been, and that she is still physically appealing and not an ugly leper. But on a metaphoric level, these lines could be read as a linguistic defense that she had nothing to do with Gloucester's death. Hoeniger states, "These words invite from us (and did from Shakespeare's Elizabethan audience) an ironic response since like the King we are convinced of her guilt and thus her spiritual leprosy" (199). The King looks away because he is aware that his wife is involved in Gloucester's death. Margaret declares that she is not a leper; therefore she is true and faithful to the King. In other words, being free of leprosy hopefully proves she provided good counsel and comfort to the King. The defense is ironic because the audience knows that she is indeed involved with Suffolk and the plot to destroy Gloucester. It is also ironic because Henry does not appear to be listening: "What? Art thou, like the adder, waxen deaf?" (76). Once again leprosy is connected to false language.

In *Anthony and Cleopatra* (1607), Shakespeare uses both leprosy and syphilis as diseases that represent a threat to society; however, in this play, the threat is connected to sexual sins, specifically to Anthony and Cleopatra's uncontrolled adulterous relationship. In Act 3 scene 10, Enobarbus asks Scarius how the sea battle goes. Scarius answers,

On our side like the tokened pestilence,
Where death is sure. Yon ribaudred nag of Egypt—
Whom leprosy o'ertake!—i' the midst o' the fight,
When vantage like a pair of twins appeared
Both as the same, or rather ours the elder,
The breeze upon her, like a cow in June,
Hoists sails and flies. (9–15)

Concerning these lines Hoeniger writes, "As in Shakespeare's time leprosy was particularly associated with Egypt, the oath is appropriate" (199). But much more is occurring in this line that a simple curse on Cleopatra. Scarius is making a distinction between two hypothetical diseases: tokened pestilence and leprosy. Scarius suggests that his navy resembles "a tokened" or spotted pestilence. This allusion could imply either smallpox or syphilis, or possibly bubonic plague. Because of Anthony and Cleopatra's adulterous relationship, it would seem more likely that Shakespeare's spotted plague is a reference to syphilis than smallpox, since that is the only disease transmitted through sexual relations. Scarius's declaration that his troops look like syphilitics underscores the idea that the sins of the leader affect the metaphoric health of the troops. Consequently, Scarius wishes Cleopatra to be infected with leprosy so that others will be protected from falling into her clutches. Scarius chooses leprosy because it is metaphorically associated with falseness, and Cleopatra has presently abandoned her troops. Both the disease she causes in her troops and the disease wished upon her are appropriate to her sins.

Scarius identifies Cleopatra as punished by leprosy, as the sin demands. Not only does Scarius state that his army looks as doomed as a plague victim, he also curses Cleopatra with leprosy because she has abandoned the troops. What Scarius implies is that those who are falsifiers and threaten the stability of the community should be stricken with a disease that identifies them as untrustworthy. Leprosy would be the appropriate disease because it marks those who threaten the stability of society. But Cleopatra is also guilty of an adulterous affair with Anthony, and because of that affair, her troops appear to represent a syphilis infection. Both leprosy and syphilis are used metonymically for the sins that each disease punishes.

One of the clearest connections between leprosy and syphilis in Shakespeare occurs in *Henry V* (1599), particularly in the humorous scenes of the tavern. In Act 2, scene 1, the audience meets Falstaff's tavern mates. Falstaff is dying. In this scene, Pistol and Nym exchange curses because Pistol has married the woman to whom Nym was betrothed. Nym wants her back and threatens Pistol, who responds to Nym's threats:

O hound of Crete, think'st thou my spouse to get?
No, to the spital go,
And from the powdering tub of infamy
Fetch forth the lazar kite of Cressid's kind,

> Doll Tearsheet she by name, and her espouse. (74–78)

While these lines are meant to be humorous, they also point to both the growing association between leprosy and syphilis and the belief that leprosy is a sexually transmitted disease. Pistol tells Nym that he cannot have Pistol's wife, called Hostess in *Henry V*, but Mistress Quickly in *2 Henry IV*. Instead, Pistol suggests that Nym should try his luck at the spital house. Hoeniger speaks to the meaning of a spittle house: "There appears to have been some distinction in usage in Shakespeare's time between hospital and spital-house or spital (spittle), the former more respectable, the latter associated with low persons and those afflicted with horrible diseases like syphilis" (25). Not only does Pistol tell Nym to take his wife from the spital house, but he also tells Nym to remove her from the powdering tub, either a reference to the sweating procedure common to sufferers of syphilis or to the tub of face powder she would need to apply to cover her sores. What is interesting is that Pistol connects a spital house and syphilis to a lazar house and Cresseid. As we have already seen, Henryson continues Chaucer's *Troilus and Criseyde* by having her suffer from leprosy. While Cresseid's punishment in Henryson's work is a result of blasphemy, Pistol's reference connects Cresseid's leprosy to sexual sins through her comparison to Doll Tearsheet, a prostitute.

Shakespeare is not the only author to connect leprosy with sex. By the time of John Ford's *'Tis Pity She's a Whore* (1633) one can see a clear connection between leprosy and sex that was not prevalent during the late Middle Ages. Near the mid-seventeenth century, one begins to see clear formulations of a sexual interpretation of leprosy that go back to Shakespeare. Considered by some to be Ford's finest play, *'Tis Pity She's a Whore* tells the tragic tale of two lovers who are brother and sister. This play contains numerous references to leprosy as a venereal disease. In the opening scene, Giovanni confesses to a Friar that he is in love with his sister. Giovanni questions, "Shall, then, for that I am her brother born, / My joys be ever banished from her bed?" (I. 39–40). The Friar responds by saying, " O, Giovanni! Hast thou left the schools / Of knowledge to converse with lust and death? / For death waits on thy lust" (I. 60–62). The Friar's counsel to Giovanni is to be penitent and on his knees "beg Heaven to cleanse the leprosy of lust / That rots thy soul" (74–75). On one level, the Friar's statement is metaphorical and connects the state of the soul to that of a disease. However, on another level the Friar connects leprosy to sexual sins, in this case incest. The Friar counsels Giovanni to do penance, and if Giovanni has "no change in thy desires, return to me" (80).

Giovanni's penance does not assuage his desires, and the reader soon learns that his sister is with child. She is quickly married to Sorenzo, a nobleman of the town, who learns that she is already pregnant. Sorenzo curses his new bride and demands the lover's name. Annabella remains faithful to her brother and Sorenzo declares that he will "drag / Thy lust-be-lepered body through the dust" (IV.iii.60). While the connection between sexuality and leprosy in the previous passage was through the sin of incest, in this passage the sexual sin is expanded to include all premarital sexual relationships, because Sorenzo is unaware of Annabella's relationship with her brother. Eventually, the Cardinal and the people of the town find out about the incest, Giovanni kills Sorenzo, and Vasques, Soranzo's servant, kills Giovanni. The Cardinal then orders Annabella to be burned alive for her sins.

Brody believes that "such references to leprosy in drama confirm that the tie between leprosy and sexuality was current not only among educated persons, but also in the popular culture generally, and the idea remained so well after the Middle Ages had ended" (192). While Brody is correct to notice that these associations were common both to educated and lay persons, it is not entirely accurate to see the connection between leprosy and sexuality as a development of the Middle Ages.

By the time of Shakespeare and Ford, leprosy began to share some of the venereal associations that were commonly connected to syphilis. But this connection does not find a lot of support in the Middle Ages, where leprosy traditionally was believed to identify those individuals who were a threat to the *status quo* of the community. When people started to become infected with syphilis in the Early Modern Period, both medical and lay persons connected moral associations common to leprosy to this new disease, primarily because it was a skin ailment. Thus syphilis was thought to represent people guilty of envy, slander, or blasphemy. As the culture became more aware of the disease and the nature of its transmission, the connection between the disease and morality shifted to sexuality. When syphilis was considered a venereal disease, leprosy also acquired some of those moral associations, primarily because leprosy was nearly a mythic disease in the sixteenth and seventeenth centuries; lepers in lazar hospitals were so few that most people in England would not have known or seen a leper. The reason leprosy did not slip completely from the common person's mind was that the Bible and literature recalled the disease. The association of sexual sins with leprosy has more to do with the interpretation of syphilis than it does with beliefs about leprosy during the Middle Ages. Furthermore, the characterization of leprosy as a sexual disease demonstrates a change in social emphasis according to which people became more concerned about individual sexuality, rather than communal relationships. In the Middle Ages, leprosy underscored sins that threaten the stability of the community. In the sixteenth and seventeenth centuries, people became more aware of what an individual was doing privately with other individuals. Therefore, there was more emphasis placed on individual sexual relationships.

Conclusion

The study of social responses to diseases such as leprosy and bubonic plague informs modern day struggles with new epidemics, such as AIDS and SARS. Leprosy is more like AIDS in that it is thought by the general society as a disease that punishes a specific individual rather than an entire group. The reason for this specificity is that AIDS, like leprosy, has limited means of transmission. For AIDS, one needs to come in contact with infected blood, semen, or vaginal fluid, unlikely in most daily experience. For leprosy, the potential for transmission is very low. Because the disease has limited means of transmission, it becomes easier to imagine the disease as a punishment for a certain type of behavior. But AIDS also has generated social responses common to bubonic plague, particularly in the interpretation of these diseases as apocalyptic punishments, and it is my belief that SARS will generate reactions more similar to the reactions to bubonic plague. In the near future, I think we will see growing prejudice toward Asian people and increasing fear that they could be carriers of the disease, much like medieval people witnessed with the Jews and bubonic plague.

It would appear that the interpretation of epidemics moves through an evolutionary process, and we can forecast how we will deal with new diseases by looking at how other cultures dealt with highly contagious diseases. Initially the disease is believed to be the end of the world and everyone becomes fearful. As a disease continues, people realize that not everyone is infected, and people begin to treat the disease according to the specificity of its means of transmission. At the heart of all these diseases lies human interpretation, particularly the comfort we feel when we construct a clear line of moral demarcation between the kingdom of the ill and the healthy.

The moral interpretation of disease began in the Greco-Roman period when Galen combined medicine with philosophy. Lacking any concept of pathogens, most people were left to wonder why certain people became ill when others did not. Doctors believed the body to be composed of four bodily humors and each humor reflected an element in the macrocosm. These humors could be influenced by outside forces, some of which included an individual's emotions and actions. Cures, at this time, required a period of moral reflection on the part of the victim because his or her actions may have contributed to an affliction. When Christianity supplanted paganism, the moral reflection on illness evolved into concepts of sin and redemption. Since most early medical learning was had in monasteries and was under the control of the church, it is no surprise that medicine and theology sought a common interpretation for disease. Consequently, when epidemic diseases struck, the only logical conclusion for clerics and doctors could be God's wrath at human sin.

Leprosy clearly demonstrated to medieval people that God could send disease as both a sign of his anger and as a warning to others concerning a leper's moral status. Because of the linguistic confusion over the Hebrew word "tsara'ath" and its subsequent translation in vulgate Bibles into "leprosy," leprosy had a clearly authoritative source for its being divinely sent. Since leprosy only affected limited numbers and was fairly difficult to contract, the sins connected with the disease seemed accurate. Further, the sins that were associated with leprosy came from the category of spiritual sins, because those sins were of greater concern than the carnal sins to the community at that time. Members of the community who held power were supposed to recognize the symptoms of the disease and remove a leper from the community so that the leper could do no further damage. In the case of leprosy at this time, the power of the disease was primarily held in the hands of God, for only God could know who had committed spiritual sins.

When bubonic plague struck society, doctors and priests applied the same interpretive structure to this disease that they had to leprosy. However, while leprosy is chronic and difficult to transmit, bubonic plague is acute and easy to transmit. Numerous people became infected with the disease, even children, who could not have committed the necessary sins for this type of punishment. In the initial interpretations, doctors and priests assumed that God was punishing all of mankind for its sin of Pride. In this sense, God moved from being the protector of a society, identifying social threats with leprosy, to a wrathful God in the process of destroying His creation. Eventually, however, the interpretation that this disease was foreboding the end of the world wore off, and people began to examine the disease from a practical and pragmatic standpoint.

Doctors provided people with information about how to protect themselves and how to treat those who contracted the disease. In this disease, one sees a movement from an interpretation of disease where God has ultimate control, to one where God still has control, but mankind can influence the number of infections and deaths. In the literature written less than one hundred years after the first outbreak, one already sees a change in the hierarchy of plague information. Information on means of transmission, prescriptions for the infected, and method of protection are placed in the forefront; whereas moral information, while still mentioned, is not the primary focus as it was in earlier plague literature.

Plague literature demonstrates a change in emphasis concerning information about the disease; syphilis demonstrates a change in behavior. When syphilis struck Europe, people interpreted the disease along the same lines as they had leprosy, owing to the notion that one skin disease must be like another. However, people of Europe quickly learned that syphilis affected the sexual organs and, therefore, was not punishing the syphilitic for spiritual sins but for carnal sins, particularly lechery. Syphilis demonstrates the movement by people to take the power of disease out of God's hands and to give people some control over disease transmission. In other words, it is difficult to know when one has committed enough spiritual sins so that one needs to be punished. When does a person act enviously enough to finally receive leprosy from God? However, if the disease is linked to carnal sins, then the power of disease transmission is more in the hands of man. If one avoids the sexual act, one can in most cases avoid the disease. Most interesting is the desire by people in the Renaissance to bring other diseases under similar control. Thus leprosy gains associations common to syphilis, even though leprosy is difficult to contract through sexual relations. The reason leprosy acquires the sin of lechery from syphilis may be because the action and reason for the disease are more tangible, more under human control.

People tend to like their diseases clearly demarcated and under human control. To see the ways people construct disease, one need only think about the modern-day hospital and the social space different groups occupy in that location. The workers, doctors, nurses, and orderlies all wear a uniform that places them into an appropriate medical hierarchy. Doctors and nurses further demonstrate medical expertise through one of the most important medical symbols—the stethoscope, usually resting around the neck of the doctor or nurse. The ill are just as clearly identified through a uniform, a short paper-like dress that leaves an open slit down the back of the patient. The ill are often placed in beds or wheelchairs, and are connected to tubes and bags, which adds to the staging of sickness. Finally, the third group is the visitors. This group is composed of the friends and families who are free to migrate from the kingdom of the well to the kingdom of the ill, as long as the stay is short. Their street clothes identify this group; they are usually given a pass that says "visitor"; and they carry an object, either flowers, food, or stuffed animals, sometimes desperately, in order to signify their citizenship in the kingdom of the well.

The social construction of the hospital demonstrates much about the way humans like to demarcate between the healthy and the ill, and the way humans like to have control over diseases that could affect them. Even though the body as text is relatively downplayed by the medical community, the general community is much more comfortable when the ill have some type of sign or symptom that clearly identifies the kingdom in which others belong. AIDS is a problematic disease in relation to these kingdoms. Like the visitor in the hospital who is free to enter the kingdom of the ill and to move freely around but cannot stay, the PWA can move freely about in the kingdom of the well, even though he or she is neither well nor able to stay for too long. The ability of a PWA to move about undetected within the kingdom of the well causes anxiety and fear, primarily because people are worried about infection and the penetration of social barriers. Most people would be perfectly content if, when someone became infected with AIDS, his or her hair would turn green and stand straight up on his or her head. The contentment that would result from this physical symbol is not based on the idea that the PWA could get immediate medical help, but rather that the rest of the society would be alerted to his or her potential transmission. The desire to have a physical symbol of the disease stems from instincts of survival and protection, and it appears to be a common human desire to label the healthy and the ill. The label is an interpretative act that attempts to both explain the disease's arrival and why the disease seeks a particular person. It is also a label that helps people gain control of the disease. Interpretation of disease gives the disease a consciousness in which it is actually seeking out a specific target, a specific human being or a specific behavior. Those who are healthy can take solace in the notion that they will not get the disease because they are not like the person who has the disease.

Women are often the target group of many of these attempts to control the disease and its means of transmission. The general anxiety that both the medieval and Early Modern societies showed toward women and women's bodies in relation to leprosy and syphilis is an anxiety that has also been expressed in our modern culture. The women-as-polluter myth is evident in medieval society in the construction of leprosy whereby a man can contract leprosy when he lies with a woman who has recently lain with a leper. The essential fear here is one of survival—the very act by which one gives life is now the act that can take life. The same social construction works for AIDS as well as leprosy, for in both cases one is believed to have received a death sentence.

Interestingly, the woman-as-polluters motif is not exclusive to a primitive cultural system or part of a society that lacks an advanced medical system. In "AIDS, Gender, and Biomedical Discourse," Paula Treichler analyzes our medical establishment's desire to keep AIDS a gay disease in the early outbreak years. As Treichler writes,

> Commitment to this view of AIDS as a male disease was so strong that when R. R. Redfield and his colleagues reported a study in the *Journal of the American Medical Association* demonstrating infection in U.S. servicemen who claimed heterosexual contact only—with female prostitutes in Germany—various attempts were made to discredit or dismiss this new evidence: servicemen, for instance, would be punished for revealing homosexual behavior or intravenous drug use; they really had gone to male

> prostitutes, and so on. If women were merely passive vessels without the efficient capacities of a projectile penis or syringe for "efficiently" shooting large quantities of the virus into another organism, the transmission to U.S. servicemen from German prostitutes must be only apparent. Indeed, one reader suggested, transmission was not from women to men but was rather "quasihomosexual": Man A, infected with HIV, had sexual intercourse with a prostitute; she "[performing] no more than perfunctory external cleansing between customers," then had intercourse with Man B; he is infected with the virus by way of Man A's semen still in the vagina of the prostitute. (207–8)

Treichler's description of this imagined type of transmission is similar to the medieval medical description of the transmission of leprosy through non-symptomatic women. Although people now have the knowledge that pathogens are transferred between human beings and cause illnesses, the myth of the woman-as-polluter remains firmly ingrained in our social consciousness. The difference between the medieval poison damsel of leprosy and the modern damsel of AIDS is that the modern relies on a different set of moral connections. The transmitters of AIDS are not simply women, but prostitutes, and the prostitutes have the ability to homosexualize men by combining their semen. Medieval doctors are not as concerned about the power of women to homosexualize men; instead, their concern is connected to the power women have to demonstrate, at best, the man's and woman's uncontrollable sexual desire, and at worst, the man's status as a cuckold. In other words, the construction of AIDS demonstrates modern fears about homosexuality, while the construction of leprosy by medieval people demonstrates their fears about fidelity.

With advent of SARS, we witness a new symbol of health or disease—the surgical mask. Many photographs of SARS outbreaks show people wearing the mask that is normally used to demarcate the healthy, the doctors and nurses in the hospital. At some level, the mask is still being used that way, as the majority of people wearing the masks are members of the healthy. However, people suffering from SARS also wear the mask as it might prevent transmission. Modern medical professionals are not even sure if these masks will prevent SARS transmission, yet many people place their faith in the mask. One wonders if the same occurred with the beak-like mask of the medieval medical doctor who wore the hood to protect himself from plague and placed vinegar or herbs in it as a way to ward off the foul-smelling contagion. Did the general population of the Middle Ages also don similar masks as we are doing today? Will we be looked at with nostalgic ignorance by later generations when the medical information about SARS becomes refined and more accurate?

As modern society continues to deal with the AIDS and SARS epidemics, people in both the medical and popular fields learn that the disease does not have a consciousness that is seeking to rid the world of a specific type of person. Too many anomalies exist of victims who are not the "sinners" the disease is supposed to be seeking. The anomalies are important because they begin to break down the clear demarcations between us and them, between the ill and the well, and between the sinners and the saints. Once this breakdown occurs, people have two choices. They can first continue to insist that the disease is God's punishment, but that He creates imperfect diseases that cannot simply attack those that are morally impure. Along this theoretical line, believers often justify God's incompetence in disease construction by saying that those who are infected but not guilty will have immediate access to heaven. The second theory is that the interpretation of the disease is wrong and that the disease can affect everyone. Eventually the majority of people choose the latter and begin to examine how the disease is transmitted and what measures can be taken to prevent further infection.

Since 1981, contemporary society has gone through the same disease evolution with AIDS, and in 2003 we are in the earliest stages of understanding SARS. Originally AIDS was labeled as a homosexual disease, thereby protecting the heterosexual community from the fear that they were at risk. When too many anomalies surfaced, the medical community announced that everyone was at risk. It was at this time that people started to search for the disease's means of transmission. Once blood and semen were identified as dangerous fluids, then the medical community constructed universal precautions for dealing with body fluids. In some ways, the precautions for AIDS and SARS are similar to the precautions medieval doctors advocated for bubonic plague. They both advocated what was at that time the accepted belief about the disease. One must remember that like the medieval doctor who did not know the exact bacteria causing bubonic plague, modern doctors still do not have a test to identify HIV; they only have a test that identifies the *antibodies* the body produces in defense of the virus. As for SARS, only recently has the coronavirus been mapped. It is possible that modern medicine could discover ideas about HIV or SARS that totally revolutionize today's interpretation of the disease.

The bubonic plague of the Middle Ages and AIDS and SARS of the modern period differ in the importance of the literary work as a means of communicating current ideas about the disease. In the Middle Ages, it appears that literature was a means by which accurate medical information could be disseminated to the general population. Through this dissemination, people protected themselves from plague and treated those infected. In our modern day, literature does not carry the same degree of valid medical information. Instead, we have social organizations that handle the role of information dissemination, including schools, non-profit organizations, and government publications. No matter what form the information takes, evolution of the interpretation of disease reflects a great deal about the fears within a society, today or a thousand years ago.

Notes

Chapter One: From *Sophrosyne* to Sin

1. See also Herzlich and Pierret, *Illness and Self in Society*, Baltimore: Johns Hopkins UP, 1987, 76–82.
2. The works of Hippocrates did not come from one author. Consequently, two opposite medical theories can find support for their beliefs within the Hippocratic Corpus. See Lindberg, 118–119.
3. For a more thorough list of writers arguing that medicine is divinely sent, see Amundsen, 135–136.
4. See also Amundsen, 133–4.
5. For a detailed discussion of medical education at Oxford and Cambridge, see Vern Bullough, "Medical Study at Mediaeval Oxford" *Speculum* 36 (1981), 600–12, and "The Mediaeval Medical School at Cambridge" *Mediaeval Studies* 24 (1962) 161–8.
6. "[C]uius quidem futuri in eo languoris et prius com adhuc communi inter fratret uita degret aspicientibus in facie eius signa patebant."
7. "multi deuota religione . . . postularent, quatinus aliquam illis particulam de reliquiis sancti."
8. "Mittens enim praefatae partem pelliculae in aquam, ipsa aqua lauit faciem suam, statimque tumor omnis qui hanc obsederat et scabies foeda recessit."
9. "gratia Dei omnipotentis, quae et in praesenti multos et in futuro cordis et corporis nostri languores sanare consueuit."

Chapter Two: Leprosy, Bubonic Plague, and Syphilis

1. For the variety of ceremonies, see Brody, 60–9.
2. See, for example, Danielle Jacquart and Claude Thomasset, 177–93.
3. In *Communities of Violence: Persecution of Minorities in the Middle Ages*, David Nirenberg also sees leprosy used as an agent of social control in France around 1341. While outside the geographical scope of this thesis, Nirenberg's work examines how rebellions against the monarchy were "cloaked by violence and accusations first against Jews, then against lepers, and finally against Jews again" (122). Accusations of leprosy became a means for government leaders to control those that threatened the established social order.

4. Some theological writers from the Continent also connect leprosy to envy. Bloomfield declares that the *Compendium theologiae* (c.1402), a pseudo-Gersonian work, makes comparisons between sins, animals and diseases. Bloomfield puts the comparison into a table for easy reference:

Sin	Animal	Disease (Latin name)
pride	lion	*corporis inflatio*
envy	dog	*lepra*
anger	wolf	*frenesis*
accidie	ass	*lethargia*
gluttony	bear	*hydropsis*
lechery	pig	*epilentia*
avarice	hedgehog	*febris* (373)

While this work is composed outside of the geographic location that this book is investigating, clearly the association between Envy, one of the spiritual sins, and leprosy is drawn in this text. It is also worthwhile to note that the author connects Lechery to epilepsy, and not to a skin disease.

5. Luke also sees this miracle as causing Jesus to withdraw from the community: "But Jesus often withdrew to lonely places and prayed" (5:16).
6. Lanfrank began his medical career in Italy as a pupil of the surgeon and teacher, William of Saliceto. Driven from Milan by the Visiconti, Lanfrank settled in France. In 1295, he was invited to Paris by Jean de Passavant, dean of the faculty of medicine, to give lectures on surgery. This appointment gave Lanfrank the time to produce his greatest work—*Chirguria Magna* in 1296 (Talbot 101). This work includes numerous medical modern sources as well as Classical and Arabic citations. *Chirguria Magna* is so important to the development of medicine in France that both Sarton and Talbot cite Lanfrank as "the father of French surgery" (784 and 102, respectively). Translated from Latin, *Chirguria Magna* became the first surgical and anatomical work to appear in the English vernacular (Sarton 1080).
7. In *Medicine and Medieval England*, C. H. Talbot argues that the earliest vernacular surgical text was published in England in 1398 (192). However, George Sarton's *Introduction to the History of Science* contends that the translation of Lanfrank's work can be accurately dated to 1380 (1080–81). I tend to believe Sarton's argument, and even if the work cannot be dated to 1380, the manuscript in which most of this work is located, *The Bodleian Ashmole*, is dated 1396, still two years earlier than Talbot's records.
8. The first edition is the quarto of 1621, although Dell and Smith use the sixth edition published posthumously in 1651. See Dell and Smith, vi.
9. See also Brody, 51–2.
10. See Hays, 64–5.
11. "qui inficitur ex coytu mulieris cum qua concubuit leperosus."
12. "Black Death" was not a term of the Middle Ages. Gottfried states that it most likely appeared in 1550 as a reference to the epidemic of 1347–51 (xvi). Medieval doctors referred to it as "pestilence" or "plague." However, for the purposes of this paper, I will use the term "Black Death," as most historians do, to refer to this pestilence of the late fourteenth century.
13. These statistics are highly controversial. Historians, like Gottfried, often attribute great weight to the Black Death concerning population reduction. For an opposing view, see Ann Carmichael, *Plague and the Poor in Renaissance Florence* (Cambridge: Cambridge UP 1986), 90–103. While historians do argue over the percentages, no one contends the plague mortality was negligible.
14. Horrox says an infected flea can live for eighty days (7).
15. See Hays, 73.

Chapter Three: Leprosy and Spiritual Sins in Medieval Literature

1. Quicksilver is also mentioned as cure for leprosy of the nose in Harley MS 2378. See Henslow, *Medical Works of the Fourteenth Century* (New York: Burt Franklin 1972), 80.
2. There are many that burn for sex.

Chapter Four: Plague as Apocalypse in Medieval Literature

1. All citations are from the C Version, edited by Derek Pearsall, *Piers Plowman* (Exeter: Exeter UP, 1978) and hereafter are listed by Passus and line number.
2. See Horrox, 84–88.
3. For the increase in bequests, see Courtenay, 709.
4. Chaucer also makes a similar statement about the Parson in the *Canterbury Tales:*

   > . . . sette nat his benefice to hyre
   > And leet his sheep encombred in the myre
   > And ran to Londoun unto Seinte Poules
   > To seken hym a chaunterie for soules,
   > Or with a bretherhed to been withholde;
   > But dwelte at hoom, and kepte wel his folde,
   > So that the wolf ne made it nat myscarie. (*Prol.* 507–13)

   While Chaucer uses this social information to characterize the piety of the Parson, Langland uses the same information to condemn the clerical order.
5. For an excellent examination of poverty in *Piers Plowman*, see David Aers, *Community, Gender, and Individual Identity* (London: Routledge 1988) 20–72.
6. For the relationship between the knight and labor laws, see Aers, *Community*, 44.
7. For an opposing view, see Zvi Razi, "Family, Land and the Village Community" in *Landlords, Peasants and Politics in Medieval England*, T. H. Aston, ed. (Cambridge: Cambridge UP, 1987), 373–5. Razi finds only a 10 percent decrease in the amount of land transferred to kin at one particular manor.
8. Beidler sees a similar level of separation between Death and the rioters. Beidler writes, "For the Pardoner's purposes his tale must clearly show that Death seizes the corrupt. The Pardoner underscores the point in a passage generally overlooked: 'the feend foond hym in swich lyvynge / That he hadde leve him to sorwe brynge' (847–48). *Because* the rioter has been living evilly, the fiend 'has leave'—presumably from God—to poison his thought in such a way that he will bring himself and his fellows to sorrow" (261).
9. The dates for the York play are much debated. Beadle notes that a document exists that asks for storage of three pageant wagons in 1376 (xv). Beadle states that a more "certain construction may be placed on a petition, dated 1399" (xv). Either way, since performance dates are uncertain, the dates of the writing of the text are also problematic.

Chapter Five: Learning to Cope with Disease

1. See also Slack, 16.
2. For information on the six non-naturals, see Siraisi, *Medieval and Early Renaissance Medicine*, 101.
3. All citations to *The Dialogue* refer to William Bullein, *A Dialogue Against the Feuer Pestilence*, eds. Mark W. Bullen and A. H. Bullen (Oxford: Early English Text Society, 1888) and is hereafter cited by page number.

4. Boring provides a nice, readable summary of a very complex work. He conveniently divides the work into nine "scenes," even though no scene markers are available.
5. For how Frye developed the term "anatomy" from one of the most famous Menippean satires, Burton's *Anatomy of Melancholy*, see Murfin and Ray, 210.
6. Antonius and Civis can also be read as symbols for Town and Country.
7. For the ability of the wealthy to avoid the stigma of plague, see Carmichael, 83–84.

Chapter Six: Leprosy and Syphilis in Early Modern Literature

1. See Siraisi, *Medieval and Early Renaissance Medicine*, 101, for a discussion of the non-naturals.
2. "pelagi terraeque labores"
3. "Illa dies, foedi ignoto tuum corpora morbo / Auxilium sylva miseri poscetis ab ista, / Donec peoniteat scelerum"
4. "luxu fastuque"
5. Citations to Spenser's *Faerie Queene* are by book, canto, stanza, and line numbers, if necessary.
6. Chew also argues that Spenser is indebted to a French "livre de miniatures" that Gower based his work on, see 37–38.
7. See J. L Lowes, "Spenser and the *Mirrour de l'omme*," *PMLA*, 29 (1914), 393.
8. For a discussion on the organization of Book II in relation to Dante, see J. Holloway, "The Seven Deadly Sins in *The Faerie Queen*," *Review of English Studies*, 3 (1952), 13–18.
9. Moreover, this brief song demonstrates the problems faced by the medical community during times of plague. Charlatans often tried to sell cure-all elixirs to the local community. There was very little social control over doctors' claims during the Middle Ages and Early Modern Period, especially during times of plague. See Rawcliffe, *Medicine and Society in Later Medieval England*, particularly her chapters on the doctor and surgeon, pp. 105–47, for a discussion of the problems of social control of the medical community.

Works Cited

Ackerknecht, Erwin H. *A Short History of Medicine*. Baltimore: Johns Hopkins UP, 1955.

Aers, David. *Community, Gender, and Individual Identity*. New York: Routledge, 1988.

———. *Culture and History, 1350–1600*. Detroit: Wayne State UP, 1992.

———. "Class, Gender, Medieval Criticism, and *Piers Plowman*." *Class and Gender in Early English Literature*. Eds. Britton J. Harwood and Gillian R. Overing. Bloomington: Indiana UP, 1994.

Amundsen, Darrel W. *Medicine, Society, and Faith in the Ancient and Medieval Worlds*. London: John Hopkins UP, 1996.

Arrizabalaga, Jon. "Facing the Black Death: Perceptions and Reactions of University Medical Practitioners." *Practical Medicine from Salerno to the Black Death*. Ed. Luis García-Ballester, Roger French, Jon Arrizabalaga, and Andrew Cunningham. Cambridge: Cambridge UP, 1994. Pp. 237–288.

———, John Henderson, and Roger French. *The Great Pox: The French Disease in Renaissance Europe*. New Haven: Yale UP, 1997.

Augustine. *On Christian Doctrine*. Trans. D. W. Robertson, Jr. New York: Macmillan, 1987.

———. *The Confessions of St. Augustine*. Trans. John K. Ryan. New York: Doubleday, 1960.

Bacon, Francis. *Essays, Advancement of Learning, New Atlantis, and Other Pieces*. New York: The Odyssey Press, 1937.

Bakhtin, Mikhail. *Rabelais and His World*. Trans. Hélène Iswolsky. Bloomington: Indiana UP, 1984.

Baugh, Albert. *A Literary History of England*. New York: Appleton Century Crofts, 1948.

Barrett, W. P., ed. *Present Remedies against the Plague, etc*. London: Shakespeare Association, 1933.

Beadle, Richard. *The Cambridge Guide to Medieval English Theatre*. Cambridge: Cambridge UP, 1994.

———and Pamela King, eds. *York Mystery Plays: A Selection in Modern Spelling*. Oxford: Clarendon Press, 1984.

Beck, Theodore R. *The Cutting Edge: Early History of the Surgeons of London*. London: Lund Humphries, 1974.

Bell, David N. "English Cistercians and Medicine." *Citeaux* 40 (1989): 139–73.

Bentley, Greg W. *Shakespeare and the New Disease: The Dramatic Function of Syphilis in* Troilus and Cressida, Measure for Measure, *and* Timon of Athens. New York: Peter Lang, 1989.

Besançon, Etienne de. *An Alphabet of Tales: An English Fifteenth-Century Translation of the* Alphabetum Narratonum *of Etienne de Besançon*. Ed. Mary Macleod Banks. London: EETS, 1904.

Beidler, Peter G. "The Plague and Chaucer's Pardoner." *Chaucer Review*. 16.3 (1982): 257–269.

Bloomfield, Morton. *The Seven Deadly Sins*. Michigan: State College Press, 1952.

Boccaccio, Giovanni. *The Decameron*. Trans. Richard Aldington. New York: Garden City, 1930.

Boeckl, Christine M. *Images of Plague and Pestilence: Iconography and Iconology* (Sixteenth-Century Essays & Studies, 53). Kirksville, MO: Truman State University Press, 2000.

Boethius. *The Consolation of Philosophy*. Trans. Richard Green. New York: Macmillan, 1989.

Boring, William C. "William Bullein's *Dialogue Against the Fever Pestilence*." *The Nassau Review* 2 (1974): 33–42.

Brody, Saul. *The Disease of the Soul: Leprosy in Medieval Literature*. Ithaca, NY: Cornell UP, 1974.

Bullein, William. *A Dialogue Against the Feuer Pestilence*. Ed. Mark W. Bullen and A. H. Auden. London: Early English Text Society, 1888.

Bullough, Vern L. *The Development of Medicine as a Profession*. New York: Hafner, 1966.

———. "Medical Study at Mediaeval Oxford." *Speculum* 36 (1961): 600–12.

———. "The Medical School at Cambridge." *Mediaeval Studies* 24 (1962): 161–68.

Burton, Robert. *The Anatomy of Melancholy*. Ed. Floyd Dell and Paul Jordan-Smith. New York: Tudor, 1927.

Cadden, Joan. *Meanings of Sex Difference in the Middle Ages: Medicine, Science, and Culture*. Cambridge: Cambridge UP, 1993.

Cambell, Sheila, Bert Hall, and David Klausner, eds. *Health, Disease, and Healing in Medieval Culture*. New York: St. Martin's, 1992.

Campbell, Ann Margaret. *The Black Death and the Men of Learning*. New York: Columbia UP, 1931.

Campbell, Oscar James. *Comically Satyre and Shakespeare's "Troilus and Cressida."* San Marino: Huntington Library, 1970.

Cameron, M. L. *Anglo-Saxon Medicine*. Cambridge: Cambridge UP, 1993.

Carmichael, Ann. *Plague and the Poor in Renaissance Florence*. Cambridge: Cambridge UP, 1986.

Chaucer, Geoffrey. *The Riverside Chaucer*. 3rd ed. Ed. Larry D. Benson. Boston: Houghton Mifflan, 1987.

Chew, Samuel C. "Spenser's Pageant of the Seven Deadly Sins." *Studies in Art and Literature for Belle da Costa Greene*. Ed. Dorothy Eugenia Miner. Princeton: Princeton UP, 1954. pp. 37–53.

Clendening, Logan, ed. *Source Book of Medical History*. New York: Dover, 1942.

Colgrave, Bertram, trans. *Two Lives of Saint Cuthbert: A Life by an Anonymous Monk of Lindisfarne and Bede's Prose Life*. New York: Greenwood, 1969.

Cooper, Helen. *Oxford Guides to Chaucer: The Canterbury Tales*. Oxford: Oxford UP, 1996.

Courtenay, William J. "The Effects of the Black Death on English Higher Education." *Speculum* 55 (1980): 696–714.

Crossgrove, William C. "Medicine in the *Twelve Books on Rural Practices* of Petrus de Crescentiis." *Manuscript Sources of Medieval Medicine*. Ed. Margaret R. Schleissner. New York: Garland, 1995. Pp. 81–104.

Curley, Michael J., trans. *Physiologus*. Austin: University of Texas, 1979.

Curry, Walter Clyde. *Chaucer and the Mediaeval Sciences*. New York: Barnes & Noble, 1960.

Dawson, W. R. *A Leechbook or Collection of Medical Recipes of the Fifteenth Century*. London: Macmillan, 1934.

Demaitre, Luke. "The Description and Diagnosis of Leprosy by Fourteenth-Century Physicians" *Bulletin of the History of Medicine* 59 (1985): 327–344.

Dols, Michael W. *The Black Death in the Middle East*. Princeton: Princeton UP, 1977.

Dyer, Christopher. *Standards of Living in the Later Middle Ages*. Cambridge: Cambridge UP, 1989.

Ebin, Lois B. *John Lydgate*. Boston: Twayne, 1985.

Ell, Stephen R. "Plague and Leprosy in the Middle Ages: A Paradoxical Cross Immunity?" *International Journal of Leprosy and Other Mycobacterial Diseases*.2 (1987): 345–350.

Ford, John. *John Ford: Five Plays*. Ed. Havelock Ellis. New York: Mermaid, 1957.

Foucault, Michel. *The Order of Things*. New York: Vintage, 1970.

Fracastoro, Girolamo. *Fracastoro's Syphilis*. Ed and trans. Geoffrey Eatough. Liverpool: Francis Cairns, 1984.

Frantzen, Allen J. *The Literature of Penance in Anglo-Saxon England*. New Brunswick: Rutgers UP, 1983.

Funkenstein, Amos. *Theology and the Scientific Imagination: from the Middle Ages to the Seventeenth Century*. Princeton: Princeton UP, 1986.

Galen. *Galen: on Respiration and the Arteries*. David J. Furley and J. S. Wilkie, ed. Princeton UP, 1984.

———. *Galen: on the Parts of Medicine, Cohesive Causes, Regimen in Acute Disease in Accordance with the Theories of Hippocrates*. Trans. Malcolm Lyons. Berlin: Akademie-Verlag, 1969.

Garbáty, Thomas. "The Summoner's Occupational Disease." *Medical History* 7 (1963): 348–358.

Getz, Faye Marie, ed. *Healing & Society in Medieval England: A Middle English Translation of the Pharmaceutical Writings of Gilbertus Anglicus*. Madison: University of Wisconsin, 1991.

Gibaldi, Joseph. *Approaches to Teaching Chaucer's* Canterbury Tales. New York: Modern Language Association, 1980.

Gottfried, Robert S. *The Black Death: Natural and Human Disaster in Medieval Europe*. New York: Macmillan, 1983.

———. *Epidemic Disease in Fifteenth-Century England*. New Brunswick: Rutgers UP, 1978.

Gower, John. *Mirrour de l'Omme*. Trans. William Burton Wilson. East Lansing: Colleagues, 1992.

———. *The Complete Works of John Gower*. Ed. G. C. Macaulay. Oxford: Clarendon, 1899.

Grant, Edward, ed. *A Source Book in Medieval Science*. Cambridge: Harvard UP, 1974.

Gray, Douglas. *Robert Henryson*. Leiden: Brill, 1979

Grmek, Mirko D. *Diseases in the Ancient Greek World*. Trans. Mireille Muellner and Leonard Muellner. Baltimore: Johns Hopkins UP, 1989.

Guy De Chauliac. *The Cyrurgie of Guy de Chauliac*. Ed. Margaret S. Ogden. London: EETS, 1971.

Harington, Sir John, Ed. *The School of Salernum: Regimen Sanitatis Salerni.* Rome: Edizioni Saturnia, 1959.

Hays, J. N. *The Burdens of Disease.* New Brunswick: Rutgers UP, 1998.

Henryson, Robert. *Robert Henryson: The Poems.* Ed. Denton Fox. Oxford: Clarendon Press, 1987.

Herlihy, David. *The Black Death and the Transformation of the West.* Cambridge, MA: Harvard UP, 1997

Hoeniger, David F. *Medicine and Shakespeare in the English Renaissance.* Newark: University of Delaware, 1992.

Holloway, J. "The Seven Deadly Sins in *The Faerie Queene*, Book II." *Review of English Studies.* 3 (1952): 13–18.

Horden, Peregrine. "Disease, Dragons, and Saints: The Management of Epidemics in the Dark Ages." *Epidemics and Ideas: Essays on the Historical Perception of Pestilence.* Eds. Terrence Ranger and Paul Slack. Cambridge: Cambridge UP, 1992. Pp. 45–76

Horrox, Rosemary, trans. and ed. *The Black Death.* Manchester: Manchester UP, 1994.

Hume, Katheryn. "Leprosy or Syphilis in Henryson's *Testament of Cresseid*?" *English Language Notes* 6.4 (1969): 242–5.

Hunt, Tony. *The Medieval Surgery.* Woodbridge: Boydell, 1992.

———. *Popular Medicine in Thirteenth-Century England.* Cambridge: D. S. Brewer, 1990.

Huppert, George. *After the Black Death: A Social History of Early Modern Europe.* 2nd ed. Bloomington: Indiana UP, 1998.

Jacquart, Danielle and Claude Thomasset. *Sexuality and Medicine in the Middle Ages.* Trans. Matthew Adamson. Princeton: Princeton UP, 1988.

Jeffrey, David Lyle, ed. *The Dictionary of Biblical Tradition in English Literature.* Michigan: Wm. B. Eerdnabs Publishing, 1992.

John Arderne. *Treatises of Fistula in Ano.* Ed. D. Power. London: Early English Text Society, 1910.

Jonson, Ben. *The Complete Plays of Ben Jonson.* Ed. G. A. Wilkes. Oxford: Clarendon, 1981.

Kealey, Edward J. *Medieval Medicus: A Social History of Anglo-Norman Medicine.* Baltimore: Johns Hopkins UP, 1981.

Kratins, Ojars. "The Middle English *Amis and Amiloun*: Chivalric Romance or Secular Hagiography?" *PMLA* 90 (1966): 347–354.

Krochalis, Jeanne and Edward Peters, eds. *The World of Piers Plowman.* University Park, PA. Pennsylvania UP, 1975.

Lanfrank of Milan. *Lanfrank's "Science of Cirurgie."* Ed. Robert V. Fleischhacker. London: Kegan Paul, Trench, Trubner & Co., 1894.

Langland, William. *William Langland's* Piers Plowman*: The C-Text.* Ed. Derek Pearsall. Exeter: Exeter UP, 1978.

Leavy, Barbara Fass. *To Blight with Plague: Studies in a Literary Theme.* New York: New York UP, 1992.

Leach, MacEdward, ed. *Amis and Amiloun.* Oxford: EETS, 1960.

Lewis, C. S. *English Literature in the Sixteenth Century, Excluding Drama.* Oxford: Clarendon, 1954.

The 'Liber de Diversis Medicinis.' Ed. Margaret Sinclari Ogden. London: Early English Text Society, 1938.

Lindberg, David C. *The Beginnings of Western Science.* Chicago: Chicago UP, 1992.

Luria, Maxwell and Richard L. Hoffman, eds. *Middle English Lyrics.* New York: W. W. Norton, 1974.

Lupton, Deborah. *Medicine as Culture: Illness, Disease, and the Body in Western Societies*. London: Sage, 1994.

Lydgate, John. *The Minor Poems of John Lydgate*. Part II: Secular Poems. Ed. Henry Noble MacCraken. Oxford: EETS, 1934.

Lyotard, Jean-François. *The Postmodern Condition: A Report on Knowledge*. Trans. Geoff Bennington and Brian Massumi. Minneapolis: University of Minnesota, 1993.

Mannyng, Robert. *Robert Mannyng of Brunne* Handlyng Synne. Ed. Idelle Sullens. Binghamton: Medieval and Renaissance Texts and Studies, 1983.

McCutcheon, Elizabeth. "William Bullein's *Dialogue Against the Fever Pestilence*: A Sixteenth-Century Anatomy." *Miscellanea Moreana: Essays for Germain Marc'hadour*. Eds. Clare M. Murphy, Henri Gibaud, and Mario Di Cesare. Binghamton: Medieval & Renaissance Texts & Studies, 1989.

McNeill, John T. "Medicine and Sin as Prescribed in the Penitentials." *Church History* 1 (1932): 41–26.

———. and Helena M. Gamer, trans. *Medieval Handbooks of Penance*. New York: Columbia UP, 1990.

McVaugh, Micheal R. *Medicine Before the Plague: Practitioners and Their Patients in the Crown of Aragon, 1285–1345*. Cambridge:Cambridge UP, 1993.

McVeigh, Terrence. "Chaucer's Portraits of the Pardoner and Summoner and Wyclif's *Tractatus De Simonia*." *Classical Folia* 29 (1975): 54–58.

Miller, Timothy. *The Birth of the Hospital in the Byzantine Empire*. Baltimore: Johns Hopkins UP, 1997.

Moore, R. I. *The Formation of a Persecuting Society: Power and Deviance in Western Europe, 950–1250*. Oxford: Blackwell, 1987.

Murfin, Ross and Supryia M. Ray. *The Bedford Glossary of Critical and Literary Terms*. Boston: Bedford, 1997.

Nirenberg, David. *Communities of Violence: Persecution of Minorities in the Middle Ages*. Princeton: Princeton UP, 1996.

O'Boyle, Cornelius. "Surgical Texts and Social Contexts: Physicians and Surgeons in Paris, *c*. 1270 to 1430." *Practical Medicine from Salerno to the Black Death*. Eds. Luis García-Ballester, Roger French, Jon Arrizabalaga, and Andrew Cunningham. Cambridge: Cambridge UP, 1994. Pp. 156–185.

Park, Katherine. *Doctors and Medicine in Early Renaissance Florence*. Princeton: Princeton UP, 1985.

Pastore, Judith Laurence, ed. *Confronting AIDS through Literature: The Responsibilities of Representation*. Urbana: University of Illinois, 1993.

Pearsall, Derek. *The Canterbury Tales*. London: Routledge, 1985.

———. *John Lydgate*. Charlottesville: University Press of Virginia, 1970.

Penzer, N. M. *Poison Damsels and Other Essays in Folklore and Anthropology*. London: Charles J. Sawyer, 1952

Platt, Colin. *King Death: The Black Death and Its Aftermath in Late Medieval England*. Toronto: University of Toronto, 1997.

Poos, L. R. *A Rural Society after the Black Death: Essex, 1350–1525*. Cambridge: Cambridge UP, 1991.

Pouchelle, Marie-Christine. *The Body and Surgery in the Middle Ages*. Trans. Rosemary Morris. New Brunswick: Rutgers UP, 1990.

The Pricke of Conscience. Ed. Richard Morris. Berlin: A. Asher, 1863.

Quétel, Claude. *History of Syphilis*. Trans. Judith Braddock and Brian Pike. Baltimore: Johns Hopkins UP, 1990.

Ranger, Terence and Paul Slack, eds. *Epidemics and Ideas: Essays on the Historical Perception of Pestilence*. Cambridge: Cambridge UP, 1992.

Rawcliffe, Carole. *Medicine and Society in Later Medieval England*. Phoenix Mill: Allan Sutton, 1997.

———. *Sources for the History of Medicine in Late Medieval England*. Kalamazoo: Medieval Institute Publications, 1995.

Richards, Peter. *The Medieval Leper*. New York: Barnes & Noble, 1977.

Riddle, John M. *Contraception and Abortion from the Ancient World to the Renaissance*. Cambridge, Harvard UP, 1992.

Rowland, Beryl. "'The Seiknes Incurabill' in Henryson's *Testament of Cresseid*," *English Language Notes* 1 (March 1964): 175–177.

Ryan, William Granger, trans. "Saint Martin, Bishop." *Jacobus De Voragine: The Golden Legend Readings on the Saints*. Volume II. Princeton: Princeton UP, 1993.

Schleissner, Margaret R., ed. *Manuscript Sources of Medieval Medicine: A Book of Essays*. New York: Garland, 1995.

Shakespeare, William. *The Complete Works of William Shakespeare*. Ed. David Bevington. New York: Bantam, 1988.

Shepard, Geoffrey. "Poverty in *Piers Plowman*." *Social Relations and Ideas*. Eds. T. H. Aston and Christopher Dyer. Cambridge: Cambridge UP, 1983.

Shoaf, R. Allen. *Chaucer's Body: The Anxiety of Circulation in the Canterbury Tales*. Gainesville: University of Florida Press, 2001.

Shrewsbury, J. F. D. *A History of Bubonic Plague in the British Isles*. Cambridge: Cambridge UP, 1970.

Simpson, R. R. *Shakespeare and Medicine*. Edinburgh: E. & S. Livingstone, 1959.

Singer, Charles. *A Short History of Medicine*. New York: Oxford UP, 1962.

———. "A Thirteenth-Century Clinical Description of Leprosy." *Journal of the History of Medicine* 4 (1949): 237–39.

Siraisi, Nancy G. "Editorial: Medieval and Renaissance Medicine: Continuity and Diversity." *Journal of the History of Medicine* 41 (1986): 392–94.

———. *Medieval and Early Renaissance Medicine*. Chicago: Chicago UP, 1990.

Skeat, Walter W. *The Complete Works of Geoffrey Chaucer: Notes to the* Canterbury Tales. London: Oxford, 1965.

Slack, Paul. *The Impact of Plague in Tudor and Stuart England*. London: Routledge, 1985.

Sontag, Susan. *Illness as Metaphor and AIDS as Metaphor*. New York: Anchor Books, 1990.

Soranus of Ephesus. *Soranus' Gynecology*. Trans. Oswei Temkin. Baltimore: Johns Hopkins UP, 1956.

Spenser, Edmund. *The Faerie Queene*. Ed. Christopher Ricks. New York: Penguin, 1978.

Strohm, Paul. *Social Chaucer*. Cambridge, MA: Harvard UP, 1989.

Sudhoff, Karl. *The Earliest Printed Literature on Syphilis Being Ten Tractates from the Years 1495–1498*. Adapted Charles Singer. Florence: R.Lier & Co., 1925.

Talbot, Charles H. *Medical Practitioners in Medieval England: A Biographical Register*. London: Wellcome Historical Medical Library, 1965.

———. *Medicine in Medieval England*. London: Oldbourne, 1967.

Temkin, Oswei. *Galenism: Rise and Decline of a Medical Philosophy*. Ithaca, NY: Cornell UP, 1973.

———. *Hippocrates in a World of Pagans and Christians*. Baltimore: Johns Hopkins UP, 1991.

Treichler, Paula A. "AIDS, Gender, and Biomedical Discourse: Current Contests for Meaning." *AIDS: The Burdens of History*. Eds. Elizabeth Fee and Daniel M. Fox. Berkeley: University of California Press, 1988.

Twigg, Graham. *The Black Death: A Biological Reappraisal*. London: Batsford, 1984.

Ward, A. W. and A. R. Waller. *The Cambridge History of English Literature*. Cambridge: Cambridge UP, 1907–1927.

Watts, Sheldon. *Epidemics and History: Disease, Power, and Imperialism*. New Haven: Yale UP, 1997.

Wenzel, Siegfried, ed. and trans. *Fasciculus Morum: A Fourteenth-Century Preacher's Handbook*. University Park: Pennsylvania State UP, 1989.

Williams, Guy. *The Age of Agony: The Art of Healing*. Chicago: Academy Chicago, 1986.

Writght, Herbert G. "Some Sixteenth- and Seventeenth-Century Writers on the Plague," *Essays and Studies*, 4 (1953):41–55.

Wright, Laurence. "'Burning' and Leprosy in Old French." *Medium Ævum* 56.1 (1987):101–111.

Zinsser, Hans. *Rats, Lice, and History: A Chronicle of Pestilence and Plagues*. New York: Black Dog, 1935.

Index